MENTAL HEALTH

A Non-Specialist Introduction for Nursing and Health Care

Edited by

ANGELINA CHADWICK
Lecturer in Mental Health Nursing, School of Health and Society,
University of Salford

and NEIL MURPHY
Lecturer in Mental Health Nursing, School of Health and Society,
University of Salford

Lantern

ISBN: 9781908625953

Lantern Publishing Ltd, The Old Hayloft, Vantage Business Park, Bloxham Rd, Banbury, OX16 9UX, UK
www.lanternpublishing.com

© 2021, Shelly Allen, Eunice Ayodeji, Lisa Bluff, Elizabeth J. Burns, Angelina L. Chadwick, Katie A. Davis, Celeste Foster, Elizabeth Garth, Will Hough, Lorna McGlynn, Neil A. Murphy, Rachel S. Price, Emma Street, Elizabeth J. Tudor and Seán Welsh

The right of Shelly Allen, Eunice Ayodeji, Lisa Bluff, Elizabeth J. Burns, Angelina L. Chadwick, Katie A. Davis, Celeste Foster, Elizabeth Garth, Will Hough, Lorna McGlynn, Neil A. Murphy, Rachel S. Price, Emma Street, Elizabeth J. Tudor and Seán Welsh to be identified as authors of this work has been asserted by them in accordance with the Copyright, Design and Patents Act 1988.

British Library Cataloguing in Publication Data
A catalogue record for this book is available from the British Library

The authors and publisher have made every attempt to ensure the content of this book is up to date and accurate. However, healthcare knowledge and information is changing all the time so the reader is advised to double-check any information in this text on drug usage, treatment procedures, the use of equipment, etc. to confirm that it complies with the latest safety recommendations, standards of practice and legislation, as well as local Trust policies and procedures. Students are advised to check with their tutor and/or practice supervisor before carrying out any of the procedures in this textbook.

Vendor	Price	Order No.
Bmns	12·29	11/21.
CLASS No.	616·89.	
ACC. No.	46045.	

Cover design by Andrew Magee Design Ltd
Typeset by Medlar Publishing Solutions Pvt Ltd, India
Printed in the UK
Last digit is the print number: 10 9 8 7 6 5 4 3 2 1

Contents

About the authors

Angelina L. Chadwick, RGN RMN BSc(Hons) PGCE MSc SFEA, is a lecturer in mental health nursing in the School of Health and Society at the University of Salford, UK. Angelina began her career as a general nurse in 1986, working in surgery. She later retrained as a mental health nurse and progressed into a variety of mental health nursing clinical and management roles in acute inpatient, older people and community practitioner areas. She moved into education as a training manager in an NHS mental health Trust, and then into higher education as a nurse lecturer in 2010. She is currently a module leader in the pre-registration degree nursing programme and teaches on both pre-registration and postgraduate programmes. Her keen interest is in physical health in mental health. Angelina has published in a variety of nursing journals and textbooks, including co-authorship of a pocket guide to mental health placements for student nurses, published by Lantern Publishing.

Dr Neil A. Murphy, RMN PhD, is a senior lecturer in mental health nursing in the School of Health and Society at the University of Salford, UK. Neil started his career as a mental health practitioner in 1980. He trained as a mental health nurse and then as a behavioural therapist, working predominantly in a community role and latterly, in his active practice, working closely with families. Neil has worked in higher education since 2002, leading and developing new programmes aimed at enhancing the quality of training offered to nurses and also to cognitive behavioural therapists and advanced clinical practitioners. Neil's main drive has been to equip as many people as possible in health care with mental health orientated skills in order to enhance care and foster client choice, empowerment and opportunity. His PhD focused on the influence of media representations on mental health practitioners and Neil has published in many nursing journals and textbooks. His publications include 'Experiences of advanced clinical practitioners in training and their supervisors in primary care using a hub and spoke model' published in *Practice Nursing* (2020; **31(8)**: 334–42).

Dr Shelly Allen, RMN/BNurs(Hons) PhD MHsc Specialist Practitioner Mental Health PGCE, is a senior lecturer in mental health nursing in the School of Health and Society at the University of Salford, UK. Shelly qualified as a registered mental health nurse, completed a Master's degree in health sciences and the Specialist Practitioner qualification in mental health at the University of Birmingham. She developed an interest in supporting people who self-harm, which led to a doctorate. Shelly combines academia and clinical practice with an honorary position while undertaking clinical training as an adult psychodynamic psychotherapist with the Tavistock and Portman NHS Foundation Trust/Northern School of Child and Adolescent Psychotherapy.

Dr Eunice Ayodeji, RMN PGCE FHEA PhD, is a lecturer in mental health nursing in the School of Health and Society at the University of Salford, and a child and adolescent cognitive behavioural psychotherapist with Bolton Community CAMHS, UK. Eunice is a child and adolescent mental health nurse who has worked in a wide variety of CAMHS, including both inpatient, forensic and community CAMHS as well as specialist CAMHS for looked-after children. She has extensive therapeutic experience with children and young people who have complex mental health and social problems and with their families and carers. She currently teaches on the undergraduate and postgraduate nursing programme. Her research interests include self-harm, emerging personality problems and depression in children and young people, and evidence-based practice. In addition to her academic role, Eunice works in a community CAMHS team. Eunice was the child and adolescent mental health nurse committee member for the National Institute for Health and Care Excellence on developing the NICE guideline for the management of depression in children and young people (2019). Since publication of the guideline Eunice continues her role at NICE as an expert in child and adolescent mental health nursing. Her recent publications include 'Depression and bipolar disorder in children and young people' in *Children and Young People's Mental Health* (2019, Pavilion Publishing).

Lisa Bluff, RMN BA(Hons) MmedSci PgDip HEPR PGDipCBP FHEA, is a perinatal training and workforce lead with Greater Manchester Mental Health NHS Foundation Trust, UK. Lisa's passion for perinatal mental health developed when studying for her psychology degree. This continued while she was working as a mental health nurse on an acute inpatient unit. Lisa then went to work as a research governance lead before joining the University of Salford in 2004. During this time she was the co-module lead for the perinatal and infant psychotherapy module and she trained in cognitive behavioural psychotherapy, working at a women's centre. Her current role is the training and workforce lead for perinatal mental health services in Greater Manchester.

Elizabeth J. Burns, RMN BNurs(Hons) MA International Addiction Studies PGCAP FEA, is a lecturer in mental health nursing in the School of Health and Society at the University of Salford, UK. Following a career in alcohol services working across a range of primary care and criminal justice settings, Elizabeth worked in public health for ten years. Here she developed both population approaches to reducing alcohol harm and individual behaviour change interventions, working on alcohol licensing policy as well as building capacity in screening and brief interventions, assessing and managing alcohol withdrawal, and safeguarding. She joined the University of Salford in 2015 and is currently a programme leader for pre-registration mental health nursing. She continues to have a particular interest in public health and is a member of the international Motivational Interviewing Network of Trainers. Elizabeth's recent public health publications include co-authorship of 'Mobilising communities to address alcohol harm: an Alcohol Health Champion approach' in *Perspectives in Public Health* (2020; **140(2)**: 88–90).

Dr Katie A. Davis, BN (Mental Health) MSc PhD PGCAP FHEA, is a lecturer in mental health nursing in the School of Health and Society at the University of Salford, UK. Katie is a registered mental health nurse with a background in older adult nursing. She has experience working in both the NHS and the voluntary sector and is passionate about working collaboratively with service users and care partners. Katie's PhD explored co-researching with people living with dementia and was awarded by the University of Manchester in 2020. She is currently a module lead in the pre-registration nursing programme at the University of Salford.

Dr Celeste Foster, BSc(Hons) RMN PGCE MA FEA Reg MBACP, is a senior lecturer in mental health and Deputy Director of the School of Health and Society Research Centres at the University of Salford, UK. Celeste is a senior adolescent mental health nurse, registered adolescent psychotherapist and academic who has been working in child and adolescent mental health since 1995. As an early career researcher, she has published in the subjects of psychoanalytic approaches to working with adolescents and their professional networks in relation to self-harm, complex psychosomatic presentations and developmental trauma. Celeste's PhD thesis focused on developing a new model of nursing practice in inpatient adolescent mental health units. She has led several multiprofessional research studies investigating effective whole-school approaches to pupils' emotional wellbeing, and effective interventions for adolescents with complex and severe mental health needs, including children with physical, neurodevelopmental and psychiatric comorbidities. A recent co-publication focuses on 'Understanding the nature of mental health nursing within CAMHS PICU' in the *Journal of Psychiatric Intensive Care* (2019; **15(2)**: 87–102).

Elizabeth Garth, Dip He RMN BSc(Hons) Dip AS PGCAP, is a lecturer in mental health nursing and programme lead for the non-medical prescribing module in the School of Health and Society at the University of Salford, UK. Elizabeth qualified as a registered mental health nurse in 1999 and worked in a variety of jobs in both acute and community settings, with her main experience in substance misuse services. Elizabeth held many clinical roles, including lead nurse for substance misuse services, developing her management and leadership skills during this time. In 2012 she completed a non-medical prescribing programme and registered as a nurse independent/supplementary prescriber with a V300 qualification, running regular prescribing clinics in substance misuse services and prison settings. She joined the University of Salford in 2015, delivering teaching, supervision and support to both pre-registration nursing programmes and post-qualifying programmes. Since 2014 she has been a member of the National Steering Group for the National Substance Misuse Non-Medical Prescribing Forum as northern region representative.

Will Hough, RMN PGCE Postgraduate Forensic, is a lecturer in mental health nursing in the School of Health and Society at the University of Salford, UK. Will has specialist knowledge and skills in deafness and forensic mental health nursing. He has held various positions within specialist deaf mental health services before working as a lecturer practitioner and moving into full time higher education in 2013. He is the university lead for the Deaf Nurse Project, supporting deaf people's access into nursing as part of the recruitment team, and he teaches on the pre-registration nursing programmes. He has a keen interest in service provision and has published on the subject of deafness and mental health.

Lorna McGlynn, RMN MSc PGCAP FEA, is a lecturer in mental health nursing in the School of Health and Society at the University of Salford, UK. Lorna is currently a mental health nursing lecturer and module leader on the pre-registration degree nursing programme. She moved into higher education in 2019, having begun her career as a registered mental health nurse in acute mental health inpatient services, working her way up to ward manager on a male acute admissions ward and psychiatric intensive care unit (PICU). She later moved into community mental health services and established a service supporting GPs and community mental health practitioners in improving the physical health and wellbeing of their service users with severe mental health conditions. Lorna later progressed into a variety of senior leadership roles, including practice and quality development lead and physical health care lead for a large NHS Trust. Lorna has a keen interest in physical health in mental health and wellbeing. Some of her publications have focused on horticultural therapy and its impact on improving depressive symptoms and can be found in the *Mental Health Nursing* journal.

Rachel S. Price, RMN Specialist Practitioner BSc(Hons) MA FHEA, is a lecturer in mental health nursing in the School of Health and Society at the University of Salford, UK. Having begun her mental health nursing career working with adults with chronic and enduring mental health problems in both ward-based and community settings, Rachel obtained her specialist practitioner award and moved into older people's care. She has held numerous senior nurse and service manager posts, particularly in the area of mental health liaison for older people. Rachel currently teaches on pre- and post-registration nurse education programmes and has a keen interest in research on vascular cognitive impairment, vascular dementia and palliative care for people dying with dementia. Rachel has published in her field of older people in various nursing journals.

Emma Street, RMN BA PGCE, is a lecturer in mental health nursing in the School of Health and Society at the University of Salford, UK. Emma began her career as a registered mental health nurse working in forensic high dependency services. She has worked in a variety of clinical roles in both community and inpatient settings, working with service users with co-existing mental health and substance misuse needs. Emma later progressed into a variety of leadership roles, most recently as a lead nurse for medicines management and non-medical prescribing. She moved into higher education in 2014. She currently teaches on both pre-registration and postgraduate programmes. Her keen interest is in mental health and substance misuse.

Elizabeth J. Tudor, SEN(G) RMN BSc(Hons) PGdip PGCE MA, is a practice education facilitator with Greater Manchester Mental Health NHS Foundation Trust, UK. Elizabeth began her career in nursing in 1977, qualifying as a state enrolled nurse working in surgery. She then retrained as a mental health nurse in 1980, specialising in older adult nursing, predominantly dementia care. In 2003 she became involved in developing the assistant practitioner role across the Trust. She qualified as a lecturer/practice educator in 2005 and was heavily involved in teaching an in-house mentorship programme and supporting mentors in practice, which has evolved into the implementation of the Nursing and Midwifery Council Standards for Student Supervision and Assessment. Elizabeth is currently working to increase student capacity across the Trust. She is a co-author of *Pocket Guides: Mental Health Placements*, published by Lantern Publishing.

Seán Welsh, RGN RMN BSc(Hons) PGCE MSc, is Head of Mental Health Nursing in the School of Health and Society at the University of Salford, UK. Seán joined the University of Salford in 2004 as a lecturer in mental health nursing and took up the post of Head of Mental Health Nursing in 2020. His clinical background as a mental health nurse centred on working with young people who experienced mental health problems. Seán is a registered general nurse, a registered mental health nurse and a registered nurse teacher with the Nursing and Midwifery Council. Seán completed his first degree in nursing studies, his Master's degree in professional practice and his postgraduate certificate in higher education research and practice at the University of Salford. Seán represents the University as a member of the influential Mental Health Nurse Academics UK group.

Abbreviations

A&E   accident and emergency (department)

ADHD   attention deficit hyperactivity disorder

AMHP   approved mental health professional

ASD   autism spectrum disorder

BPC   British Psychoanalytic Council

CAMHS   child and adolescent mental health services

CBT   cognitive behavioural therapy

COPD   chronic obstructive pulmonary disease

CPA   Care Programme Approach

CRHTT   crisis resolution and home treatment team

CQC   Care Quality Commission

EIS   early intervention (in psychosis) service

EIT   early intervention (in psychosis) team

GMMH   Greater Manchester Mental Health NHS Foundation Trust

GP   general practitioner

IAPT   Improving Access to Psychological Therapies

MUS   medically unexplained symptoms

NCCMH   National Collaborating Centre for Mental Health

NCISH   National Confidential Inquiry into Suicide and Safety in Mental Health

NHS   National Health Service

NICE   National Institute for Health and Care Excellence

NMC   Nursing and Midwifery Council

OCD   obsessive–compulsive disorder

ONS	Office for National Statistics
PHE	Public Health England
PICU	psychiatric intensive care unit
PPP	postpartum psychosis
PRN	when required (pro re nata)
PTSD	post-traumatic stress disorder
RCN	Royal College of Nursing
SMI	severe mental illness
UNCRC	United Nations Convention on the Rights of the Child
WHO	World Health Organization

Introduction

Mental health is something that we all possess alongside our physical health. However, in health care services, funding and the focus for debate are commonly attached to the more tangible physical ('seen and understandable') aspects of health. It is easier to recognise someone who has collapsed with a heart attack or someone who is bleeding due to an injury than it is to recognise someone who is depressed or someone who is paranoid. Therefore, those with a 'seen and understandable' illness are more likely to have access to services than those whose illness is not as apparent or understood. Over recent years you will have become aware of the increase in awareness of mental health issues and problems, through the media and those you come across in physical health care services.

You will have become aware that, as we live longer and make lifestyle choices that can have an impact on our physical and mental health, people are also more prone to more than one illness; this is known as comorbidity or multimorbidity. An example of this would be a young person diagnosed with type 1 insulin-dependent diabetes who becomes depressed at the thought of the restrictions this could pose on their life; or another person struggling with a long-term illness such as psoriasis becoming increasingly anxious about leaving their home and becoming agoraphobic. As a result, there has recently been a call for 'parity of esteem' in health care policy and literature. This means there is a drive to raise the importance, awareness, services and funding of mental health care to that of physical health care. So, you may ask, what has all of this got to do with this new mental health textbook? Well, the answer lies in those patients you will be nursing. Many will have both physical and mental health problems due to lifestyle choices, inequalities in access to health care services and living longer.

The Nursing and Midwifery Council (NMC), as a professional body, sets standards of proficiency and competencies to guide the pre-registration training and development of qualified nurses, to ensure that they are knowledgeable and skilled to nurse the patients in their care. The review of these pre-registration nursing standards (NMC, 2018a) has emphasised the need for all fields of practice to be aware of the practice and utility of skills in other fields of the health care service. So just as mental health nurses need to be knowledgeable and skilled in recognising physical health problems in patients with mental health problems, the same principle applies to non-mental health nurses, to adult, learning disability, and children and young people's nurses, and even to midwives, all of whom need to know about mental health problems. In a bid to increase the knowledge and skills of non-mental health nurses through teaching within our higher education institute, we, as a team of mental health academics and practitioners, have developed this textbook. It is aimed at non-mental health nurses, to support development in your knowledge, understanding and skills to recognise, support and signpost someone with an emerging or known mental disorder.

The chapters of this textbook focus on the many different dimensions of mental health and illness across the age continuum. *Chapter 1* looks at what mental health and illness are and the differing terms used, as well as the interplay with physical health. In *Chapter 2* we explore the different approaches and theories around mental illness, to develop your knowledge about their origins and how these differ from the medical model. *Chapter 3* focuses on the important communication skills required to support someone in mental crisis. *Chapter 4* considers many of the common diagnosable mental disorders and aims to make them understandable. *Chapter 5* explores mental health in early life, i.e. children and young people, and discusses therapies and services available to this group. *Chapter 6* examines mental health in adulthood and the services available to those individuals. *Chapter 7* moves on to mental health in later life, discussing the mental health conditions of older adults and exploring the interventions, practice and services available. *Chapter 8* considers legal and ethical aspects when supporting those with mental health problems, as well as your role and responsibilities as a professional in this area. Finally, *Chapter 9* examines risk in mental health, as well as stigma and labelling, which contribute to the ignorance and fear people have towards those with a mental illness.

The chapters have been written by experienced mental health nurses working in education, with further contribution from experienced practitioners. These individuals have a wealth of knowledge, experience and expertise, and have published extensively in many different nursing journals and now in their chosen chapter(s). Given the bank of their clinical experiences we felt it prudent to permit the authors to use varying terms when referring to patients, clients and/or service users depending on their specialist areas. Similarly, in reference to those with mental health problems they use the terminology from their practice areas, for example mental health difficulties, mental conditions and others. We hope that from reading the text, undertaking the activities and reflecting on what you have learnt you will develop professionally and ultimately be a more holistic practitioner.

Angelina Chadwick
Neil Murphy

Chapter 1
Mental health and wellbeing

Angelina Chadwick and Lorna McGlynn

LEARNING OUTCOMES

By the end of this chapter you should be able to:

1.1 Define mental health and wellbeing

1.2 Discuss the mental health continuum

1.3 Explore mental distress, mental illness and mental health problems

1.4 Examine the relationship between mental and physical health

1.5 Describe ways to promote mental wellbeing and good mental health.

1.1 Introduction

Mental health is everyone's business. One in four adults will experience a mental health condition in any given year (NICE, 2019b); one in eight children aged between 5 and 19 years will have had at least one mental disorder, with many continuing into adulthood (NHS Digital, 2018). As a health care student or practitioner on placement or working in a non-mental health care environment, you are highly likely to come across patients in your care who have or will develop mental health problems.

To understand what is meant by mental health problems, you first need to be able to differentiate between the many terms used in mental health. Therefore, this chapter will explore the many connotations of mental health, prompting you to consider patients in your care as well as your own mental health. Differences between mental health, wellbeing, distress, problems and illness will all be examined. We will also explore the relationship between mental and physical health, which is fundamental for those of you practising in non-mental health environments. Finally, health promotion will be discussed, focusing on promoting good mental health.

1.2 Mental health and wellbeing

There are many definitions attributed to mental health and wellbeing, sometimes referred to as positive mental health. The World Health Organization (WHO, 2018b)

defines *mental health* as not just the absence of a mental disorder but *a state of wellbeing*, where everyone realises their own potential and copes with the normal stresses of life, while working productively and contributing to their community. Mental health essentially centres on a person's emotional, psychological and social wellbeing; in short, the way they think, feel, act, make lifestyle choices and cope with the stresses of everyday life. It is worth noting that everyone has mental health just as we have physical health, and it should not be viewed in a negative way.

It is important to remember that mental wellbeing is not dependent on mental health status (Department of Health, 2011a). Someone who has been diagnosed with a mental health problem can have good wellbeing. An example would be a person who has been diagnosed and has a history of depression being mentally well and functioning at work. Conversely, someone who has not been diagnosed with a mental health problem may find it difficult to cope with adverse life events. The example here is where a person is struggling to cope following a marital separation – this will usually be a temporary state of distress and at some point they will revert to a state of mental wellbeing.

Maintaining good mental health and wellbeing can be influenced by many factors, such as the way we think, our social networks, diet, exercise and sleep. Having good mental health and wellbeing is just as important as having good physical health, since poor mental health can have a direct impact on a person's physical health and vice versa. Maintaining good mental health, even in the first few years of life, is associated with better long-term mental, physical and social outcomes in adult life (McDaid, Hewlett and Park, 2017). Hence, we can see the importance for the development and continuation of good physical health of taking care of a person's mental health from an early age.

Mental wellbeing protects the body from the impact of life's stresses and traumatic events and enables the adoption of healthy lifestyles and the management of long-term illness. Mental wellbeing is related to, but not the same as, the absence of mental ill health as defined earlier (Faculty of Public Health and Mental Health Foundation, 2016). Improved mental health and wellbeing are associated with a range of better outcomes for people of all ages and backgrounds. These include improved physical health and life expectancy, better educational achievement, increased skills, reduced health risk behaviours such as smoking and alcohol misuse, reduced risk of mental health problems and suicide, improved employment rates and productivity, reduced anti-social behaviour and criminality, and higher levels of social interaction and participation (Department of Health, 2011a).

ACTIVITY 1.1

Reflecting on the definition above, how would you define mental wellbeing? What does mental wellbeing mean to you?

1.2.1 What can have an impact on mental health and wellbeing?

Poor mental health and wellbeing can lead to more serious longer-term mental health problems, which may in turn affect a person's quality of life. As with our physical health, if a person does not look after their mental health, they can suffer consequences leading to longer-term mental health conditions which are harder to treat and recover from. There are many factors that can contribute to a person's overall mental health and wellbeing, including:

- poverty
- unemployment
- social isolation
- poor housing
- violence
- abuse
- trauma
- lifestyle choices
- lack of social connections.

For example, a person's lifestyle choices can have a positive or negative impact on their mental health; studies have shown that some healthy lifestyle choices, such as more frequent physical activity, non-smoking and regular social activities, are related to improvements in mental health (Velten *et al.*, 2018).

ACTIVITY 1.2

Review the lifestyle factors identified above and consider how nurses can support a person to improve these areas to positively promote the person's mental health and wellbeing.

1.2.2 Mental health as a continuum

Mental wellbeing and mental illness are opposing concepts, with many degrees of mental health in between; this can lead to some stress and distress being mistakenly viewed as mental illness. When we are happy, physically healthy, sleeping and performing well, then we may be 'flourishing' (see *Figure 1.1*). It is important to realise that, at times, our everyday lives can be hampered with feelings of unhappiness resulting from conflict at home, problems at work, worries about money, problems with children and concerns over our physical health, to name but a few examples. But these feelings and stresses can be a part of normal everyday life, and we may move along the continuum, from 'flourishing' to 'going OK', still relatively well and managing to cope with life. Moving further along this continuum, at times we experience longer periods of stress and distress caused, for example, by the loss of employment, the diagnosis of a long-term condition or losing someone we are close to through bereavement. These life events may result in a degree of mental distress or even a period of becoming mentally unwell and we may be perceived as 'unsettled'.

Mental illness or having a mental health condition sits at the opposite end of the continuum to 'flourishing' and is said to be when a person cannot cope or experiences extreme emotions such as anger, excessive anxiety, etc.; they may even become suicidal. The person should recover to some degree and become mentally well again, hence the continuum.

Flourishing	Going OK	Unsettled	Mental health condition
Normal functioning	Average functioning and few incidents of distress	Occasional and time-limited periods of stress with some impact on functioning	Signs and symptoms that are frequent, distressing and have significant impact on daily functioning

Figure 1.1 *The mental health continuum (after Beyond Blue, 2019).*

It is important to understand that there are many theories and models widely published about the causes of mental illness, and these will be discussed in *Chapter 2*. However, you need to understand that a person can be mentally well while experiencing some day-to-day stresses.

ACTIVITY 1.3

Draw a line like the mental health continuum in *Figure 1.1* and plot where you think you are on it when you think about how you feel day to day over a period of a typical week or a month.

1.2.3 Mental distress, mental illness and disorder, common mental health problems and severe mental illness

So far, a few different terms have been mentioned interchangeably, such as mental distress, mental illness and common mental health problems; but what do these all mean?

Mental distress can be described as the emotional response a person experiences at some point in their life and will usually be brief. This is important to consider in non-mental health care environments when you come across patients with physical health problems. For example, you may have a patient who was admitted for exploratory bowel surgery but returns from theatre with a temporary colostomy. This would probably result in some distress and psychological unrest for the patient and they may require support. However, they may not necessarily develop a mental health problem or require a referral to specialist mental health services. As stated earlier, we will all experience differing levels of mental distress from both expected and unexpected life events, but following a period of distress and with the support of those around us we revert to a state of mental health.

Mental illness and *mental disorder* are overarching terms used interchangeably to describe common mental health problems and severe mental illness and mental health problems. Mental illness comprises a broad range of problems, with different symptoms and generally characterised by some combination of abnormal thoughts, emotions, behaviour and relationships with others (WHO, 2019b).

The term *common mental health problem* is used when referring to commonly experienced mental disorders where a person can still manage to function in their everyday lives. For example, at any given time one in six adults have a diagnosis of anxiety and/or depression (National Clinical Audit of Anxiety and Depression, 2019). An example of this is a patient visiting you as a practice nurse for monitoring of their type 2 diabetes. You observe over recent visits that the person is less communicative and seems more withdrawn, but when questioned they say they are still managing to go to work. You establish from the patient's history that they have had a previous episode and treatment for depression, at which point you raise your concerns with the patient and they agree to see their GP.

Conversely, *severe mental illness* (SMI) is a frequently used phrase referring to severe and enduring mental illness. It is generally accepted to have three elements (Working Group for Improving the Physical Health of People with SMI, 2016):

- diagnosis: a diagnosis of schizophrenia, bipolar disorder or other psychotic disorder is usually implied
- disability: the disorder causes significant disability
- duration: the disorder has lasted for a significant duration, usually at least two years.

For the purposes of this textbook, we will generally use these terms as follows:

- **mental health problems** or **conditions** or **illness** or **difficulties** – used when discussing all forms of mental disorder
- **common mental health problems** – used to discuss problems such as anxiety, depression, etc., that are experienced commonly
- **severe mental health problems** or **severe mental illness** – used to discuss disorders that require specialist mental health service input and support, such as schizophrenia, bipolar disorder, etc.

ACTIVITY 1.4

Make a list of the mental health problems (both common and severe) that you are aware of and think about the patients in your area. How many have you seen with any from your list?

1.3 The relationship between mental health and physical health

For many years, the excess mortality rates in people with mental health problems have been widely documented. Brown *et al.* (2010) found that people with a severe mental illness die up to 20 years younger than their peers in the UK. In 2016, the Mental Health Taskforce reported that physical and mental health are closely linked and that people with severe and prolonged mental illness are at risk of dying on average 15 to 20 years earlier than others, highlighting one of the greatest health inequalities in England (Mental Health Taskforce, 2016). The risk factors for physical and mental health problems commonly overlap, and the effect of social and environmental determinants on physical health can have a profound influence on resilience. This explains why the physical health of people with severe and enduring mental illness is often poor (Oken, Chamine and Wakeland, 2015).

ACTIVITY 1.5

Think about the possible interactions between a person's mental health and physical health. Why do you think there is a 15- to 20-year increased mortality rate in a person with a mental health condition?

There are many factors contributing to the inequalities in mortality rates in people with mental health conditions, particularly those with severe mental health problems. Many of these factors can be attributed to modifiable determinants of ill health such as smoking, poor diet, lack of physical exercise, alcohol and substance misuse. People with a severe mental illness are also four times more likely to die from respiratory disease than the general population (Brown, Inskip and Barraclough, 2000; Cohen and Phelan, 2001), which can be attributed to the fact that rates of smoking in this group are considerably higher than in the average population (NICE, 2015). Furthermore, 19% of people with severe mental illness will develop hypertension, compared with 15% of the general population (Hennekens *et al.*, 2005), and there is a higher prevalence of type 2 diabetes among people with severe mental illness than in the general population (McIntyre *et al.*, 2007). These increases can be linked to the fact that people with psychosis tend to lead sedentary lives, eat less fruit and vegetables and are more likely to be obese, contributing to poor physical health (Gray, Hardy and Anderson, 2009). However, it is not just lifestyle factors that contribute to increased mortality rates; for example, some antipsychotic medications are known to cause weight gain, leading to hyperlipidaemia and diabetes (Ashworth, Schofield and Das-Munshi, 2017).

ACTIVITY 1.6

Reflecting on the lifestyle factors contributing to the increased mortality rate of people diagnosed with severe mental illness, identify what you as a nurse could do to support a person to improve their physical health.

Unfortunately, there are many barriers to receiving medical treatment for people with mental health conditions. Robson and Gray (2007) reported that there is a lack of awareness, understanding and education among health professionals and that people with mental health conditions are often unaware of what screening and services are available for their needs. Other major obstacles in accessing health care for this group of people include getting to their GP's surgery, long waiting times, communication problems, stigma, discrimination and confidence issues. Both patients and health professionals may interpret symptoms of physical disease, possibly even red-flag symptoms, as just another manifestation of their severe mental health problem, a process known as 'diagnostic overshadowing' (see *Section 3.2.5*). Owing to these significant barriers, symptoms of life-threatening conditions such as cancer may be missed, resulting in the condition going undiagnosed or untreated (Hippisley-Cox *et al.*, 2007).

1.3.1 Physical health and mental health

People with long-term physical health conditions who frequently use health care services are more likely to be experiencing mental health problems such as depression and anxiety, or dementia in the case of older people. As a result of these comorbid problems, their long-term condition and the quality of life they experience can both deteriorate markedly (Naylor *et al.*, 2012). Seventeen physical health conditions have been associated with increased suicide risk, with brain injury having one of the highest risks. In addition, having multiple physical health conditions increases this risk further (Ahmedani *et al.*, 2017). Various research studies have identified a number of physical health conditions, such as cardiovascular disease, diabetes, multiple sclerosis, musculoskeletal disorders, liver disease, kidney and end stage renal disease, COPD/bronchitis/emphysema, asthma, cancer and strokes, that can all be associated with depression (National Collaborating Centre for Mental Health (NCCMH), 2010).

For example, a cancer diagnosis can result in mental health problems – this has been found to be the case in 3% of patients with lung cancer and 28% of patients with brain cancer (Krebber *et al.*, 2013). Research evidence consistently demonstrates that people with long-term physical conditions are two to three times more likely to experience mental health problems than the general population (Naylor *et al.*, 2012).

ACTIVITY 1.7

Patients and practitioners tend to focus on the physical symptoms in consultations (Coventry *et al.*, 2011).

Consider the above statement in relation to your own area of practice. Why might practitioners only focus on a patient's physical health symptoms; what might the barriers be for non-mental health professionals?

There is growing evidence that addressing the psychological and mental health needs of people with long-term conditions more effectively can lead to improvements in both mental and physical health (Naylor *et al.*, 2012). Psychological therapies such as cognitive behavioural therapy (CBT) can help people to adapt to chronic physical illness and to develop resilience (Sage *et al.*, 2008). Around 40% of people with depression and anxiety disorders also have a long-term physical health condition. Approximately 30% of people with a long-term physical condition and 70% of those with medically unexplained symptoms (MUS) also have mental health comorbidities such as depression and anxiety. However, these common mental health problems can affect a person's ability to self-care and self-manage their long-term condition, which in turn can increase complication rates and disability, decrease quality of life, increase health care use and cost, and increase risk of early death (Egede and Ellis, 2010).

Combining pharmacological and brief psychological interventions has been shown to reduce symptoms of anxiety and depression and improve quality of life and physical functioning (Von Korff *et al.*, 2011; Whooley and Unützer, 2010). The Improving Access to Psychological Therapies (IAPT) programme in Britain has recruited and trained a workforce capable of delivering the psychosocial elements of integrated care across a wide range of long-term physical and mental health conditions. Focusing on a person's physical condition can be a barrier to recognising underlying mental health problems, so the IAPT service aims to ensure that people with long-term physical conditions and MUS have the same access to NICE-recommended psychological therapies as other people. This developing service aims to bring together mental and physical health care providers so they can work in a coordinated way to achieve the best outcomes for all people, irrespective of diagnosis (NCCMH, 2018a).

1.4 Promoting mental health and wellbeing

Just like physical health, there are areas health professionals can focus on to support people to look after their mental health and wellbeing. It is important to remember that good mental health starts with good maternal health and parenting. Social and biological influences on a child's life start before conception and continue into early years development. Therefore, as a midwife, health visitor, children's nurse or adult nurse, the mental health and wellbeing of those you support and care for are your responsibility and your concern.

Evidence gathered by the Foresight Mental Capital and Wellbeing Project (2008) suggested that a small improvement in mental wellbeing could help to decrease some mental health problems and help people to flourish.

In 2019, Public Health England updated their wellbeing and mental health guidance for health care professionals (PHE, 2019c), identifying six core principles that health professionals should work towards:
- meeting the patient's mental health and wellbeing needs
- helping to identify those at risk of poor mental health
- preventing mental health problems from developing or worsening
- preventing suicide

and when working with patients who have existing mental health problems, they can:
- ensure that their physical health needs are met
- support their social needs.

Health care professionals have a key role in providing advice and support to enable people to improve their mental health and wellbeing. This can be done using various evidence-based approaches, such as motivational interviewing, coaching and providing brief advice on various health-related issues, such as alcohol, smoking, obesity and physical inactivity, using the Making Every Contact Count (MECC) approach (PHE, 2018a).

'Five ways to wellbeing' is a widely used range of behavioural change approaches that aim to help people maintain good health and wellbeing. Evidence suggests there are five steps we can all take to improve our mental wellbeing (Aked *et al.*, 2008):

- **connect** – connect with the people around you
- **be active** – find an activity that you enjoy and make it a part of your life
- **keep learning** – learning new skills can give you a sense of achievement and a new confidence
- **give to others** – volunteering at your local community centre can improve your mental wellbeing and help you build new social networks
- **be mindful** – be more aware of the present moment, including your thoughts and feelings, your body and the world around you. This approach is used by organisations such as the NHS as a framework or a method for improving health and wellbeing and can be used by health professionals to begin conversations about a person's overall health and wellbeing.

Mental health, wellbeing and physical health are intrinsically linked, and health professionals can play a key role in promoting and supporting people to maintain good mental health and wellbeing by using a variety of interventions and approaches. It is known that, in populations with higher levels of mental wellbeing, fewer people develop mental health problems (Department of Health, 2011a). Therefore, it is important that nurses focus on the whole person during the assessment process, the planning of patient care and the delivery of any interventions, to ensure that the person's physical and mental health are equally addressed.

1.4.1 Your own mental wellbeing

Having good mental wellbeing is equally significant for all health care professionals. The Nursing and Midwifery Council (NMC) outlines in the Code of Conduct (NMC, 2018b) that nurses must act as role models to others (20.8) and maintain a level of health to carry out their professional role (20.9). This means that, to role-model your professional practice, you must be physically and mentally well to be able to undertake your responsibilities. It has been well documented that nursing as a profession is stressful (Ford, 2014; Jones-Berry and Munn, 2017), a situation that has a negative impact on nurses' physical and mental health. This can result in high levels of absenteeism from the workplace, which can in turn have a negative effect on colleagues' health and the delivery of quality patient care. The Royal College of Nursing has developed a guide to help nurses manage stress, *Stress and You: a guide for nursing staff* (RCN, 2015), which may be useful to review in terms of recognising and managing your stress levels to avoid the risk of developing physical and/or mental health problems.

ACTIVITY 1.8

Reflecting on your own health and wellbeing, list the strategies you use to promote both your physical and mental health.

Physical health	Mental health

CHAPTER SUMMARY

Key points to take away from *Chapter 1*:
- ☑ Mental health and wellbeing are influenced by early life experiences.
- ☑ Mental health is not merely the absence of illness and can be experienced along a continuum of mental health.
- ☑ Mental and physical health are inextricably linked, so patients must be holistically cared for, with all their needs identified and addressed.
- ☑ Health promotion is needed to prevent further complications for the people with long-term mental and physical conditions you are caring for and to maintain your own mental wellbeing as a practising health care professional.

Questions

Question 1.1	Develop your own definition of mental health and wellbeing based on what you have now learnt. *(Learning outcome 1.1)*
Question 1.2	Describe the mental health continuum by providing some examples. *(Learning outcome 1.2)*
Question 1.3	Describe the differences between mental distress, mental illness and mental health problems. *(Learning outcome 1.3)*
Question 1.4	Describe the relationship between physical and mental health. *(Learning outcome 1.4)*
Question 1.5	List five ways in which you can promote good mental health. *(Learning outcome 1.5)*

FURTHER READING

Nash, M. (2014) *Physical Health and Well-Being in Mental Health Nursing: clinical skills for practice*, 2nd edition. McGraw-Hill.

Norman, I. and Ryrie, I. (eds) (2018) *The Art and Science of Mental Health Nursing: principles and practice*, 4th edition. Open University Press.

Chapter 2
Approaches to mental health

Seán Welsh

LEARNING OUTCOMES

By the end of this chapter you should be able to:

2.1 Describe a range of approaches used in modern mental health care

2.2 Discuss the nurse's role and contribution to these approaches

2.3 Recognise the principles on which these approaches are based

2.4 Identify the evidence and theory that underpin these approaches.

2.1 Introduction

Modern approaches to mental health care encapsulate a broad range of underpinning theories, philosophies and perspectives.

This chapter will build on the concepts of mental health and wellbeing that were introduced in *Chapter 1* by identifying and introducing the key contemporary approaches to mental health care. The chapter will also encourage you to think about how these approaches can be applied to your own practice. Try to think of the term 'mental *health*' as a positive term or statement, i.e. maintaining or seeking to achieve mental health; it is not a euphemism for 'mental *illness*'.

ACTIVITY 2.1

Think about the people you have met, known, loved and admired over the course of your life. Did any of those experience mental illness? Did those people fit the stereotype of a 'mad' person? How did mental illness affect the individual?

There is a strong argument to say that most mental health conditions or symptoms that are associated with a diagnosis of a mental illness cannot be cured, as such. There is, however, considerable evidence that many symptoms of mental illness can be treated, controlled or reduced (Isaacs, Sutton and Beauchamp, 2020; Weiland, 2020).

The first steps in addressing concerns about mental ill health usually involve consultation with a suitably trained mental health professional such as a mental health nurse, psychologist, occupational therapist, social worker or psychiatrist.

Often these professionals will work together with the individual as part of a multidisciplinary team to help provide personalised, holistic care and treatment to address all the individual's needs (Hammond and Hammond, 2019).

ACTIVITY 2.2

Make a list of the different mental health services you are aware of. Think about who provides each service, where it takes places and what its aims are.

Are these services based in hospitals, mental health units or the community? Are they provided by specialist mental health practitioners, volunteers, generic health or social care professionals, religious leaders or by other mental health service users?

Among the broad range of mental health professionals, there is an equally broad range of approaches that these practitioners use to seek to understand and treat mental illness. The next section of this chapter will highlight some of these approaches.

2.2 The biomedical approach to mental health

The biomedical approach is perhaps the most well established and probably the most recognisable approach in mental health care in the Western world. The biomedical approach, sometimes known as the disease model or illness model (Kiesler, 2000), considers mental health conditions such as schizophrenia, substance dependency or major depression almost exclusively in terms of biologically based disorders of the brain. This approach emphasises the use of pharmacological treatment to address biological abnormalities (Deacon, 2013). The biomedical model places less emphasis on social and psychological aspects of mental disorders in favour of biological approaches, diagnosis and classification (Engel, 1977).

ACTIVITY 2.3

Make a list of mental health problems or mental illnesses that you are aware of. Working through your list, note whether you think each of your entries may have been caused by a biological illness, or whether there are other factors that may be involved.

Emil Kraepelin (1856–1926) is often referred to as the founder of modern psychiatry. Kraepelin considered psychiatry as a scientific, medical specialism and he drew a clear distinction between his mentally ill patients and 'normal people' (Steinberg, Carius and Fontenelle, 2017). Kraepelin is particularly influential as regards the classification of mental illnesses; his definitions in the mid-1890s continue to shape our understanding of affective disorders (such as bipolar disorder) and schizophrenia (Kendler and Jablensky, 2011).

The biomedical model has also influenced the language we use in relation to psychiatric medication or 'psychopharmacology': the medications we now refer to as antipsychotics were originally called major tranquillisers, and anxiolytics were previously known as minor tranquillisers (Moncrieff, 2008).

ACTIVITY 2.4

Chapter 1 established that one in four adults will experience a mental health condition in any given year (NICE, 2019b), and therefore it is likely that you or a friend or family member have experienced a mental health condition.

With this in mind, how do you feel about the distinction between a 'mentally ill patient' and a 'normal person'?

What impact could this distinction have had on stigma and on disclosure of symptoms of mental ill health?

The concept of psychiatric diagnosis became more popular from the early to mid 1970s (Double, 2003) with the introduction of diagnostic criteria and the Diagnostic and Statistical Manual of Mental Disorders (DSM) (American Psychiatric Association, 2013). Diagnostic criteria were specifically developed to address criticism about the unreliability of psychiatric diagnosis and of labelling patients using the biomedical model (Blashfield, 1984).

2.3 Behavioural approaches to mental health

Although it is fair to say that behavioural approaches are not as common or as popular as they once were, it is important to acknowledge their influence on our current perspectives and understanding of human psychology and behaviour (Michie *et al.*, 2018).

Behavioural approaches utilise practical techniques to change or stop behaviours that may be considered problematic (sometimes referred to as *maladaptive* behaviours) and replace them with more positive, beneficial or *adaptive* behaviours. Consider how behavioural approaches underpin a range of behaviour change endeavours in modern life, such as smoking cessation programmes or weight management protocols (Maisano, Shonkoff and Folta, 2020; Peckham *et al.*, 2017).

ACTIVITY 2.5

Can you identify and list what might be considered the positives and negatives of a biomedical approach to mental health?

Does your list have more positives or more negatives?

If you consider the biomedical approach from the point of view of a health professional, a service user or a family carer, does that perspective change whether something might be considered a positive or negative aspect?

Behavioural approaches are grounded in the principles of behaviourism – the concept that we are shaped by our environment (Skinner, 1938). Behavioural approaches are highly action focused and aim to help individuals develop new, positive behaviours to reduce, change or stop existing negative or unwanted behaviours (Patey *et al.*, 2018).

Behaviourism is a facet of psychology that focuses on observable human behaviour, as opposed to a Freudian belief that our unconscious mind drives our behaviour (Bollas, 2018). Behaviourism considers the conditions that cause us to produce and sustain (classical conditioning), reinforce (operant conditioning) or imitate behaviour (modelling) (Skinner, 1985). The foundations of behaviourism are rooted in three underpinning tenets: that our personalities are determined by our prior learning, that behaviour can change over the life course and that behavioural changes are usually triggered by changes in environment (Mitchell, 2019; Woolard, 2010).

You may well be familiar with 'Pavlov's dogs' and the concept of classical conditioning, where Ivan Pavlov (1849–1936) found that dogs could be conditioned to salivate at the sound of a bell, which they associated with feeding, even on subsequent occasions when food was not present. John B. Watson (1878–1958) further developed Pavlov's ideas and theories and became known as the father of behaviourism.

An emotional response to an experience can be positive or negative, and a bad experience can also produce a physiological response of fear or anxiety. The thought or prospect of being exposed to a similar negative experience may evoke the emotional and physiological response without actually being exposed to the stimulus.

ACTIVITY 2.6

Think of an experience that made you nervous or anxious; for some students this could be speaking in front of a group, or perhaps sitting an unseen examination paper.

Now try to think about your physiological response at that time: did you experience 'butterflies in the stomach', sweaty palms, increased heart rate, increased respiration rate? You may, even now, feel some of these symptoms simply at the thought of invoking memories of a difficult experience.

2.4 Psychological approaches to mental health

Psychological approaches cover a range of attitudes and methods that seek to draw on social and environmental factors in order to develop an understanding of how an individual's patterns of behaviour and experiences are linked, and subsequently to use this understanding to reduce the individual's distress.

Psychological approaches can be considered distinct from the biomedical approach (May, Cooke and Cotton, 2008). Psychological approaches challenge the biomedical assumption that a chemical abnormality is the root cause of mental ill health, that psychological phenomena can be reduced and allocated to a diagnostic category, or that they can be successfully managed predominantly by pharmaceutical interventions (Deacon, 2013).

There are several popular psychological models, including psychoanalytic, cognitive behavioural, existential–phenomenological humanistic, and family systems approaches. Psychological approaches share assumptions regarding human nature, how behaviour can go wrong and how interventions can correct or prevent what could be considered to be abnormal behaviour (Peterson, 2012).

Stickley and Freshwater (2008) provide a clear and helpful illustration of the distinction between the psychological and medical approaches by using the example of an individual who as a child lost a parent in a road accident and subsequently experiences despair and low mood in adulthood after a relationship breakdown. A medical perspective could consider these experiences to be the symptoms of clinical depression and treatment could include the prescription of antidepressant medication (American Psychiatric Association, 2013). A psychological perspective, however, may consider these phenomena to be indicative of a grief state from the loss of the adult relationship as well as unresolved emotional pain stemming from the childhood bereavement. Rather than pharmacological interventions, psychological treatment could centre on emotional and psychological exercises to try to understand, cope with and work through loss-related experiences and behaviours (Stickley and Freshwater, 2008).

2.5 Cognitive approaches to mental health

Cognitive approaches encapsulate several approaches to mental health that focus on what we might describe as *internal* phenomena such as memory, decision-making, attention and perception (Jung *et al.*, 2014; Vuilleumier, 2005). Looking at mental health in this way draws on the assumption that our brains actively process sensory information in a similar way to how a computer processes data.

Building on the foundation of this concept, cognitive approaches assert that, having processed sensory information, our brains subsequently examine the intricate processes linking sensory stimulation and our responses. In short, cognitive approaches emphasise the way we interpret/think about situations and how such interpretations/thoughts then affect resultant behaviour. After all, it is not the situation or thought that necessarily causes us problems; it is the interpretation/ thought we have related to it.

Cognitive behavioural therapy (CBT) was developed by Aaron Beck in the 1960s and is an example of a popular cognitive approach to mental health care (Beck, 1967). CBT is a means to explore our thoughts in relation to life events and to uncover how unhelpful thought patterns can be associated with maintaining rather than resolving troublesome emotional and physiological states (Turton, 2015).

2.6 Psychodynamic approaches to mental health

Psychodynamic therapy is part of a range of available treatments and, like all psychological therapies, aims to help people try to make sense of their experiences and alleviate psychological distress. Psychodynamic therapy is built on the notion that making sense of our experiences and developing an understanding of the link between what we do, how we feel and how we think can help contribute to recovery.

Psychodynamic therapy draws on the concept that our sense of self and of our worth, our understanding of others and the world around us, and how we cope are founded on learning from our most important relationships and from significant adults in our childhood. We carry internalised versions (object relations) of these that continue to influence and to be shaped by the relationships and experiences we go on to have through our adolescence and adulthood (Bateman and Holmes, 2005).

Psychodynamic therapy sessions can often seem less structured than other kinds of therapeutic approach. The individual is encouraged to speak freely about whatever is on their mind, even if it does not seem as though it is related to the agreed goals of therapy. This is because in this type of work all communication is understood to carry important information embedded within it about how the individual perceives themselves and others and how they make sense of their experiences. This means that it can be a helpful approach for people who struggle to take part in more structured interventions (Bell, 2006).

The role of the therapist (who may also be a mental health nurse) in psychodynamic therapy includes:

- *Keeping a focus on both direct and indirect expression of emotion:* working to put into words the therapist's understanding of what the individual communicates through words, non-verbal communication, their physical appearance, behaviour and the feelings that get stirred up in the therapist (projective identifications). The aim is to enable the individual to become aware of the full range of their feelings, including contradictory feelings, feelings that are troubling or threatening and unconscious feelings that initially may not be recognised as their own.
- *Noticing and exploring* themes and patterns in thoughts, feelings, self-concept, relationships and life experiences, as well as attempts by the individual to avoid distressing thoughts and feelings (defence and resistance).
- *Utilising the therapy relationship* to help illustrate and understand patterns in other interpersonal relationships (past and present, internal and external) that are repeated within the therapy relationship and to help the individual consider the impact of these patterns on their life and sense of wellbeing.
- *Keeping a developmental focus:* being mindful of the influence of early experiences on our experience of relating to the present – how thinking about the past can shed light on current psychological difficulties and help us loosen its grip (Lemma and Young, 2010).

2.6.1 Ways in which psychotherapy can help

Psychotherapy (Shedler, 2010) can help people to:
- make sense of their experiences
- distinguish between past, present and future, and internal and external reality, encouraging testing of present reality and experimentation with new ways of coping and understanding
- reduce coping strategies (defences) that are risky or that get in the way of development (e.g. self-harm or avoidance)

- build up tolerance to strong emotions and changes in mental state, and a capacity to bear and think about these, rather than having to act them out.

Psychotherapy is often criticised for having too strong a focus on what is wrong inside the person. Therapy needs to acknowledge the realities of the individual's context by being careful not to challenge too hard or too quickly defences that are there for good reason (Midgley and Kennedy, 2011).

Psychodynamic ways of working are usually most effective as part of a multidisciplinary team approach, contributing to assessment, shared formulation (understanding or explanation) and approaches to managing the difficulties the individual is encountering.

There is a particularly strong link between psychodynamic therapy and nursing; in fact, mental health nursing is fundamentally psychodynamic in nature. Nurses work to provide emotional containment of distress, to make emotional and psychological sense of what service users are doing and to restore purpose. This includes nurturing, challenging habits and defences, and developing an active capacity in the individual to be able to see beyond their current difficulties, guiding them with plans and strategies for moving forward. All of this is based on the idea that it is within the quality of the relationships we make that change occurs (Flynn, 1998).

Communicating by stirring up strong feelings in others is one our earliest means of relating to others – our survival as babies depends on it. We all rely more heavily on it during times of illness and stress, and adolescents, caught in uneven power relationships with adults, are particularly prone to returning to this way of communicating. It can be for the purpose of communication, ridding ourselves of difficult feelings, defending ourselves from others or preserving something good. In a psychodynamic model, the strong feelings aroused in us as practitioners by the service users we work with are not to be put aside but can be reflected on as an important source of information about how the service user is feeling, or about the issues underlying some of the more challenging or risky things that they do. This can complement nursing expertise to help work through behaviours and dynamics that can sometimes, understandably, leave staff groups feeling stuck and frustrated (Bradley, 1998).

2.7 Humanistic approaches to mental health

Humanism is a psychological approach that emphasises the uniqueness of human existence – that we all have different views on life and on our experiences within it (Stickley and Freshwater, 2008). Mental illness is often seen as something that happens to other people (Porter, 1987), perhaps with an unspoken implication that it is a result of some form of social or genetic deviancy or weakness. However, when we consider that each week one in six people in the UK experiences a common mental health problem (McManus *et al.*, 2016) we can see that, in fact, the truth lies much closer to home.

Barnham and Hayward (1991) emphasise the importance of recognising personhood in people who experience mental illness so that we empathise with the individual and avoid their dehumanisation, or what Porter (1987) refers to as non-identity or the non-person. In working with and caring for individuals who experience mental illness, humanism indicates that it is critical that we view their symptoms or medical diagnosis as important components of their life, but not as the *only* aspect of their life.

ACTIVITY 2.7

Humanists tend to refer to the people they work with as 'clients' rather than patients. What do you think the reason for this is?

Carl Rogers was an eminent humanist and is credited as the founder of the highly influential client-centred approach to counselling. Humanism seeks to provide the conditions to enable the individual to overcome challenges and to 'grow' and achieve self-actualisation by considering how they make meaning from experiences. In this way, the individual is not expected to comply with a medical expert's instructions (as with the biomedical model). Rather, the approach places the individual as the expert in their own life experience.

Rogers (1957) identified three core elements that are necessary for positive development in all relationships and that provide the necessary conditions within a therapeutic relationship, for example between a nurse and a client. The core conditions are:

- respect
- empathy
- genuineness.

Respect in the context of humanism is sometimes known as unconditional positive regard – this is the concept of aiming to achieve and actively demonstrate a purely respectful attitude towards the individual we are working with. This is a key foundation in developing a trusting therapeutic relationship, particularly since we know that individuals who have a diagnosis of a mental illness are often subject to prejudice and stigma (Knaak, Mantler and Szeto, 2017; Morgan *et al.*, 2018).

Empathy in the context of humanism is the attempt to understand another's experiences, concerns and perspectives and to express this understanding with the intention to help (Hojat, DeSantis and Gonnella, 2017). Empathy is not the assumption that, because we may have had a similar life experience, such as a bereavement, we know how the individual must be feeling. Rather, it is the attempt to shift our frame of reference to that of the individual and truly try to see through their eyes (Elliott *et al.*, 2011).

Genuineness, sometimes also referred to as congruence or transparency, was considered to be the most important core condition by Rogers (Worth and Proctor, 2020). In the context of humanism, congruence refers to being authentic and breaking down the façades that come between individuals by developing the therapeutic relationship – Rogers referred to this as accurately matching experience with awareness (Rogers, 1957).

2.8 Psychosocial approaches to mental health

Psychosocial approaches, often referred to as psychosocial interventions or PSIs, focus on psychological and social factors and how these may affect symptoms of mental illness, functioning, social inclusion and quality of life (Barbui *et al.*, 2020). Psychosocial interventions are a key aspect of the mental health nurse's role and they follow the principles of personal recovery – working in partnership with individuals to enable them to experience a fulfilling and valued life (Mutiso *et al.*, 2019). Zubin and Spring's (1977) stress–vulnerability model underpins the psychosocial approach, whereby both the impact of stress on the individual and their predisposing vulnerabilities are recognised as factors in their health.

Psychosocial interventions encapsulate a range of different therapeutic models and techniques, including cognitive behavioural therapy, dialectical behavioural therapy and compassion-focused therapy. Psychosocial interventions can be considered a person-based intervention, because in addition to addressing primary symptoms, they also seek to address secondary experiences that arise because of the mental health problem (Turton, 2015).

Psychosocial interventions are sometimes described as non-pharmacological interventions (Barbui *et al.*, 2020). However, pharmacological interventions are recommended as concurrent treatment with psychosocial interventions in the treatment of some disorders, e.g. psychosis (NCCMH, 2014).

Collaborative and holistic assessment is a key aspect of the nurse's role in delivering an effective psychosocial approach. It is also important that the nurse is appropriately trained in the specific psychosocial interventions they provide and engage in clinical supervision to maintain high standards and clinical efficacy.

2.9 Trauma-informed approaches to mental health

Trauma-informed approaches to mental health care stress the need to recognise and accept the impact that trauma can have on individuals, and they have seen a significant increase in influence and popularity in recent years (Kezelman and Stavropoulos, 2012; Tebes *et al.*, 2019), with the claim that trauma is as closely linked to mental ill health as smoking is to cancer (Franks, 2016).

Childhood experiences are associated with brain development and function (Bremner, 2002). Positive experiences are linked to an increase in intra-brain connectivity, whereas traumatic experiences correlate with the suppression of neural pathway development (Fan *et al.*, 2011).

Elliott *et al.* (2005) developed ten principles of trauma-informed care, emphasising the need for interventions and services to be respectful, welcoming, safe and helpful to survivors, while acknowledging the obstacles and unique needs of those who seek help. The following list highlights the ten principles.

Trauma-informed services:

- recognise the impact of violence and victimisation on development and coping strategies
- identify recovery from trauma as a primary goal
- employ an empowerment model
- strive to maximise the individual's choices and control over recovery
- are based on a relational collaboration
- create an atmosphere that is respectful of survivors' need for safety, respect and acceptance
- emphasise the individual's strengths, highlighting adaptations over symptoms and resilience over pathology
- have the goal of minimising the possibilities of re-traumatisation
- strive to be culturally competent and to understand each individual in the context of their life experiences and cultural background
- solicit consumer input and involve consumers in designing and evaluating services.

These principles provide a positive and encouraging structure, but Cutcliffe, Travale and Green (2018) highlight the current experience of mental health care by many service users as one that lacks warm therapeutic relationships, choice or respectful interactions. Using a trauma-informed approach begins with, but also is fundamental to, the enabling nature of the person-centred nurse–client relationship (Muskett, 2014).

CHAPTER SUMMARY

Key points to take away from *Chapter 2*:
- ☑ The biomedical approach views mental health conditions almost exclusively in terms of biologically based disorders of the brain and emphasises the use of pharmacological treatment.
- ☑ Behavioural approaches utilise practical techniques to change or stop behaviours that may be considered problematic (*maladaptive*) and replace them with more positive (*adaptive*) behaviours.
- ☑ Psychological approaches argue that mental health difficulties and presentations are also linked to social and environmental factors and cannot be explained in purely biological terms. These approaches tend to focus on the interpretation of thoughts, feelings and behaviours and the meaning made of them.
- ☑ Psychological interventions can be commonly viewed as a talking approach in which a person experiencing mental ill health can be helped to look at their emotions and actions related to their thinking and to identify ways of both coming to terms with them or altering them in some fashion.
- ☑ Trauma-informed approaches highlight the impact of experiences (especially as a child) of traumatic incidents. They explain some of the brain changes that may occur (especially in younger people), but focus on the person, contextualising the experiences and building change on a structured set of principles.

Questions

Question 2.1	Describe the psychological approaches commonly used in modern mental health care. *(Learning outcome 2.1)*
Question 2.2	Discuss the contribution the nurse offers in the utility of psychological approaches with people experiencing mental ill health. *(Learning outcome 2.2)*
Question 2.3	Can you list any principles on which psychological approaches are based? *(Learning outcome 2.3)*
Question 2.4	Identify at least one psychological approach and detail the evidence and theory that underpin it. *(Learning outcome 2.4)*

FURTHER READING

Black, D., Newman, N., Harris-Hendricks, J. and Mezey, G. (1997) *Psychological Trauma: a developmental approach*. Gaskell.

van der Kolk, B.A. (2015) *The Body Keeps the Score: mind, brain and body in the transformation of trauma*. Penguin.

Chapter 3
Communicating, relating and providing support

Elizabeth Tudor and Angelina Chadwick

LEARNING OUTCOMES

By the end of this chapter you should be able to:

3.1 Explore the key principles when communicating and relating to someone experiencing mental health problems

3.2 Discuss concepts around the core conditions, knowledge and skills required to support individuals with mental health problems

3.3 Examine the values, personal and professional behaviour that nurses bring to their practice

3.4 Recognise challenging behaviour and conflict and respond appropriately.

3.1 Introduction

This chapter will explore the communication and interpersonal skills required that are fundamental to providing support in everyday mental health nursing practice. These skills are transferable to any field of nursing practice and will be explored here in the context of supporting individuals with mental health needs within a non-mental health environment.

3.2 Communication skills

In your nursing practice you will be aware of the importance of communication skills, both verbal and non-verbal, which are essential interpersonal skills. There are a variety of verbal skills, such as:

- *closed questions*, which simply seek a yes or no answer and a limited verbal response
- *open questions*, which generally use 'what', 'why', 'when', for a more in-depth response
- *funnelling*, which is a technique of starting with an open question and then probing further with more focused questions to narrow down the issue
- *clarifying approaches*, which seek to clarify a point by asking a further question

- *summarising*, where you repeat something back to a person using the person's own words
- *paraphrasing*, which is similar to summarising, but in paraphrasing you use your own words.

Non-verbal communication also includes a variety of elements, both from the person and the nurse:

- *Eye contact* is vital to engage with the person. This must be appropriate – for example, you should avoid staring, as this might appear confrontational. Cultural aspects and norms should also be considered here.
- *Body posture* reflects how the person may be feeling. If they are open and leaning forward that could indicate that they are approachable. Alternatively, if they are closed, with crossed arms and legs, this may indicate that they do not wish to engage.
- *Proxemics* is about personal space and what is acceptable in an interaction, as opposed to an invasion of someone's personal space.
- *Behaviour* could indicate how an individual is feeling – for example, whether they are relaxed and settled or restless and rocking.

Non-verbal communication can sometimes be an indicator that the person may not actually be how they verbally report they are. For example, when you ask someone how they are feeling, they may say that they are fine, but their non-verbal responses include poor or avoidant eye contact, low tone of voice, closed posture and hunching over and sitting away from you. These non-verbal responses indicate that the individual may be in distress or even depressed, even though they state that they are 'fine'.

When communicating with people, particularly those with mental health problems, it is important to observe their verbal responses and non-verbal cues as well as your own. If you do not appear receptive or are rushed, this may deter a person from telling you how they are feeling or what their stresses are. You must not only be observant of others' non-verbal cues but also congruent in your own verbal and non-verbal communication. Be mindful of your professional communication skills as a nurse. Think about adopting non-verbal approaches such as SOLER (Egan, 1975) or SURETY (Stickley, 2011), since people often mirror health care practitioners' behaviours. This is particularly important when considering conflict, which will be discussed later in this chapter.

3.2.1 Appropriate language

Part of effective communication is to avoid technical terminology and to be mindful of your language. Nursing language has over time assumed a medical terminology and diagnostics sometimes known as labelling. Patients are sometimes referred to by their illness or presenting problem, for example the MI (myocardial infarction) in bed 3. This type of language should be avoided. Although diagnosis may be important to patients, in terms of understanding why they feel or behave in a certain way, this approach can leave the person feeling depersonalised. For the nurse it veers away from a person-centred caring approach, since a patient should not be defined by their illness. This is crucial when considering patients in general adult care who have a comorbid mental health problem – for example, someone with a diagnosis of schizophrenia. Referring to them as being 'a schizophrenic' can be perceived as stigmatising. Instead, we should adopt a person-centred approach by referring to the person as they wish to be referred, while still being aware of their health care needs.

3.2.2 Trust

Trust is crucially important when developing a therapeutic relationship. Patients are placed in a very vulnerable position and rely on nurses to be honest, competent, knowledgeable and dependable, and to accept the person for who they are. Patients put their trust in nurses and need to feel safe in their relationship, so that they can share their worries and anxieties, trusting the nurse to act professionally and non-judgementally regardless of the content of any information shared. Therefore, nurses must act with honesty and integrity at all times (NMC, 2018b), as once trust has been breached it is very difficult to re-establish the relationship. It is important to follow through with any commitments. If you have agreed to do something for or with a patient you must ensure that you are consistent in your approach and not go back on your word. If you are unable to fulfil a request, then you should go back to the patient to explain the reasons why. Treat your patients with respect and uphold their human rights.

3.2.3 Compassion

Compassion is one of the 6Cs and is a value and behaviour that is fundamental to delivering care through relationships based on empathy, respect and dignity (NHS Commissioning Board, 2012). Compassion is particularly important when supporting individuals with mental health problems, since at times they can be treated disrespectfully. An example of this could be when a patient has been admitted with pneumonia but they also have a diagnosis of schizophrenia and are a heavy smoker. Some nurses may see the mental illness and their behaviour of heavy smoking as contributing to their physical ill health; or they may fear the person's mental illness, reacting in a judgemental manner or avoiding caring for the person. This is stigmatising and uncompassionate. As a nurse you need to empathise with the person who is physically ill, whatever their mental illness and lifestyle choices may be, and provide compassionate non-judgemental care. This may be challenging for you, but all patients must be treated in a compassionate manner.

3.2.4 Stigma

Stigma refers to the social consequences of negative attributions about a person based on a stereotype. It presumes that individuals with mental health problems cannot be understood and lack social competence and that they are dangerous (Pilgrim, 2019).

The media does not always portray mental health in a positive light, inaccurately representing an individual with a mental health problem as unpredictable, aggressive and potentially violent, which is misleading and stigmatising. Negative views of mental illness can be held by people in all walks of life and this includes health care professionals and family members (Haddad and Haddad, 2015).

In consequence, some health care staff may experience a perceived fear of dealing with patients with underlying mental health problems in a physical health care setting. However, Pilgrim (2019, p. 169) noted that 'the vast majority of those with a psychiatric diagnosis are no more violent than those without a diagnosis'. One in four individuals will suffer from mental health problems in their lifetime, some facing discrimination based on certain diagnostic labels. Individuals with anxiety and depression may be viewed as needing to 'pull themselves together' (Haddad and Haddad, 2015). Yet many with the right support can manage their depression or anxiety and do not require hospital admission. A person with schizophrenia may be seen as aggressive, yet they are far more likely to be a victim of violence than to be violent towards another person. A person with dementia can face discrimination and social rejection and be considered a burden to society. Yet many can find a good quality of life with the support of family and friends.

3.2.5 Rapport

Rapport is pivotal in the development of a therapeutic relationship as well as in all aspects of nursing practice, since we undertake personal care procedures such as bed bathing, we insert catheters and we need to ask intimate questions about bowel habits or end of life issues. All these intimate interactions require a level of rapport within a trusting professional relationship. In mental health nursing, rapport enables nurses to relate to, collaborate with and care for patients, as well as allowing us to ask important questions about medication side effects such as sexual dysfunction, or about someone's suicidal thoughts. Rapport can be defined as 'a connection between two people where they talk on the same wavelength, sharing humour, pain and sorrow' (Sharples, cited by Brooker and Waugh, 2013, p. 208). To be effective practitioners, we need a level of rapport in order to do this, which is more than just a social aspect. Sharples outlines levels of rapport as follows:

- **Level 1: No rapport** – strangers who have just met and neither need nor want to know each other.
- **Level 2: A connection creating good communication** – people are maintaining the effort to understand each other socially, professionally. They are finding out about each other and using interpersonal skills effectively.
- **Level 3: Excellent communication**, relaxed and easy, where both parties sense a physical closeness – people feel involved, and that the other person really knows them and that they can share anything.

People you nurse who have physical health problems may require psychological support or even referral to mental health services, should they struggle to cope with recent life-changing surgery or some bad news, such as a poor prognosis. Therefore, rapport must be established with the person first, in order to be able to observe changes and ask appropriate questions through your interactions. An example of this could be when you are part of a district nursing team and are visiting a patient who has been having a leg ulcer dressed daily. On this visit, your fifth, you observe the patient to be quiet and distracted. You have limited time allocated for the visit but have noted the patient's lack of communication. You have two options – leave as planned to get to your next visit, or use your communication skills, perhaps with an open question, and rapport to allow the patient to tell you how they are feeling: *'You seem quieter today than usual, how are you feeling?'*.

This second approach indicates to the patient that you have observed a change in them and are seeking to find out what the matter is.

Another important aspect when considering rapport is the possibility of 'diagnostic overshadowing', which signifies a situation in which health care practitioners attribute behaviour or symptoms to a particular illness or diagnosis, to the exclusion of any other underlying cause. Diagnostic overshadowing happens frequently with mental health patients. For example, when someone presents at A&E with chest pain but has a long history and diagnosis of anxiety and depression, the health care practitioners may attribute the chest pain to anxiety rather than investigating a physical cause such as a cardiac event.

Diagnostic overshadowing can be challenging for nurses in a non-mental health setting, who also may attribute a change in symptoms or behaviour to the patient's physical diagnosis, which can be detrimental to patient care. For example, you may have a patient who has been admitted for investigations into an underactive thyroid. They have a long history of major depressive disorder, but you respond to their needs based on their medical diagnosis, when their deterioration could be attributed to their depression. You need to consider the effect such actions related to overshadowing may have on your relationship with the patient and how they try to make sense of the care you are providing. Establishing rapport with your patients can help to avoid diagnostic overshadowing.

3.3 Core conditions

You were introduced to Carl Rogers in *Chapter 2*, who developed a construct of three core conditions for an effective therapeutic relationship: unconditional positive regard (acceptance, respect), genuineness (honesty, trust) and empathic understanding (communication). Here we explore the core conditions further in relation to the therapeutic relationship.

3.3.1 Acceptance/unconditional positive regard

A fundamental aspect alongside rapport in the development of the therapeutic relationship is unconditional positive regard. As a nurse in a non-mental health environment, you will need to be able to demonstrate unconditional positive regard for all your patients. There may be someone who misuses alcohol who is an inpatient on a medical unit for liver problems. The challenge for you will be to accept this person when you know that their alcohol addiction is perpetuating their liver problems. In your communication with them you will need to put aside any judgements, as you support their recovery.

ACTIVITY 3.1

Jane is a 17-year-old girl who has been admitted for observation following a near fatal overdose and feels very upset about her unsuccessful attempt to take her own life. She appears angry with the staff caring for her and feels she is not worthy of being saved.

What behaviour may Jane exhibit?

Describe your feelings for Jane. How can you demonstrate unconditional positive regard?

3.3.2 Congruence/genuineness

As one of the core conditions, congruence highlights the importance of a nurse being genuine and real, to enable a more trusting relationship to develop with a patient (Rogers, 1957). More recently the condition of congruence has been called 'genuineness' (Cassedy, 2014). A willingness to engage with a patient can help in building up a trusting therapeutic relationship. Genuineness does not mean that the nurse is required to express all their feelings, but it is important to ensure that your body language and expressions are congruent with your actions. This means not feeling and thinking one thing while saying something different. For example, although well-meaning, the nurse may say: *'Don't worry, everything will be fine'*. Yet the nurse's facial expressions may contradict their verbal comments and indicate that they are not being fully truthful; thus the patient may perceive that this nurse is hiding something.

Nurses can foster trust by being consistent in their words and actions. The emphasis is on being yourself and not putting up a 'front' and hiding behind a professional façade (Cassedy, 2014). How you approach patients can have an impact on the individual's outcome, and effective communication is key. Therefore, it is important to recognise that many patients may be feeling anxious and frightened by their unfamiliar experience, and those with underlying mental health issues may find that their experience intensifies their emotional response. A culture of warmth and genuineness that is open and honest can foster a trusting therapeutic relationship whereby the patient may begin to feel safe enough to communicate.

Another way to be genuine is showing interest in everyday things, such as the person's family, hobbies and so on, during nursing interventions, steering them away from focusing on their illness. In addition, don't be afraid to use a little humour, as this can go a long way, provided it is used in an appropriate, sensitive and respectful manner. Laughter is thought to have many positive benefits for patients, in that it can reduce stress and can help the patient relax.

Being non-judgemental can be challenging, particularly if a patient's psychiatric history conflicts with your own values and beliefs. Therefore, the notion of congruence is not always easy to achieve (Freshwater, 2005). This is especially notable when there is a power imbalance in which nurses may have knowledge and information that is not available to the patient. This means that nurses may have to think about their responses and draw on their own self-awareness.

3.3.3 Self-awareness and empathy

Empathy, according to Rogers (1957), is a deep desire to understand the experience of another human being and is central to all forms of helping relationship. To provide effective humanistic care, health care staff should have a healthy sense of self. Self-awareness is a process of reflection on our knowledge of ourselves and it involves the self-management of our thoughts and feelings towards a patient. Self-awareness is made up of three components: emotions (affective), actions (behavioural) and thoughts (cognitive). It is essential that we think about our own thoughts and feelings about situations that can occur in practice.

For example, if you feel negatively towards patients who self-harm, this may affect your interactions with them. Individuals can be stigmatised for their behaviour and some nurses feel uncomfortable empathising with a patient who has self-harmed, viewing them as 'wasting their time' or 'a nuisance' and their action as 'a selfish act for attention'. They may be seen as individuals who do not deserve the same compassion as people who are physically ill (Cassedy, 2014). Not all self-harm behaviour is linked to suicidal ideation – it may be an activity that releases tension and does not signal a desire to die (Pilgrim, 2019).

By the same token, a patient who has attempted to take their own life may not be relieved that they have been saved by others; they may feel that they made a logical decision to resolve a situation and be very angry at the outcome. Yet, there may be diverse and complex issues that have contributed to their self-harming behaviours that need further investigation and support. Being empathic is an attempt to see the person's life through their own eyes and to acquire an understanding of how they feel. It demonstrates that you have genuine concern. Empathy is thought to have a positive outcome in reducing anxiety and worry. Nurses are aware of the popular expressions 'putting themselves in someone else's shoes' and 'caring for someone as if they were their own'. Some examples are listed below of patients' articulation of nurses being empathic:

Patient: *'He didn't need to say anything, he was there for me at my time of need.'* (This is known as therapeutic silence.)

Patient: *'I don't know her very well, but she finds time to listen and get to know me and she appears genuinely interested.'*

Patient: *'The nurse sensed I needed to talk about death and dying following my cancer diagnosis.'*

Patient: *'She took time to explain the procedure and when I got distressed, she reassured me it was normal to feel anxious and went through what would happen again, she made me feel at ease.'*

In addition, although at times controversial, touch can be a nursing intervention to demonstrate compassion, empathy and kindness during care, such as a touch of the hand or a reassuring hug. However, nurses need to be aware of the cultural needs, preferences and beliefs of their patients. For example:

- a person with short-term memory problems leading to confusion may respond well to therapeutic touch that conveys non-verbal empathy
- for some Muslims, touch is only permissible if there is a valid reason for it.

Nurses also need to be aware that patients may have a history of being abused and that touch may not be appropriate. Therefore it is important to ensure always that the patient gives their consent.

Nurses may struggle to provide time to listen and to empathise with patients, particularly in busy medical or surgical environments when they have large workloads and time is of the essence. Many acute hospitals now have mental health liaison teams located on site who can provide extra support.

3.4 Therapeutic relationships/therapeutic alliance

A core part of a nurse's role is building up therapeutic relationships with a patient (also known as a therapeutic alliance). As already described in this chapter, the fundamental principles of the therapeutic relationship are *genuineness*, *empathy*, *respect* and *trust*. Two further principles are:

- *active listening* – this is a skill that requires you to concentrate and fully listen to what a person is saying in order to respond and show understanding of what has been discussed
- *confidentiality* – you must protect the patient's information and explain to them how their information can be shared and who with.

These principles should continue through the duration of the therapeutic relationship, which is based on a helping relationship in which the nurse uses their skills to address the health care needs of the patient.

Peplau (1952) identifies five sequential phases in the interpersonal relationship: **orientation, identification, exploitation, resolution and termination**.

Orientation – this phase is where the nurse and the patient come to know each other, first impressions are made, and the nurse promotes trust and relieves any anxieties with the patient. This is where a history will be taken, and the patient can ask questions and clarify any worries or concerns. At this point it might be helpful to name who will be supporting the patient. Active listening will help the patient move onto the next stage.

Identification – the patient relates to the nurse and the nurse begins to get an understanding of the patient's situation. At this stage a level of rapport between the nurse and the patient is beginning, and then a more mutually agreed plan of care is developed. For example, a patient may worry that their antipsychotic medication may be missed if they have to spend five days in hospital following surgery, which could have a detrimental effect on their mental health. Can the person still receive their medication? They may have already discussed this with their community nurse prior to admission and may provide information to inform their plan of care. The named nurse can gain consent (in order to adhere to the principle of confidentiality) from the patient to speak with their community nurse to see whether that person can attend the ward to administer the medication and discuss any detrimental effects that the surgery may have had, to ensure that the patient's needs are met. The nurse must listen to the patient's concerns with respect and empathy and act on their needs. This will contribute to the patient feeling they can trust the nurse to care for them.

Exploitation – interventions are mutually agreed and supported. It is important for patients to feel that they are involved in their own care.

Resolution – the requirement to prepare for the termination phase – this is the point at which the nurse and the patient identify that the mutually agreed actions have led to the therapeutic relationship nearing an end. The patient may not require any further input, as the situation has been resolved; or they may need repeated admissions for corrective surgery and long-term support, both physically and psychologically.

Termination – the end of the therapeutic relationship; each nurse will bring their own experience as this is a valuable time to review the experience and bring closure.

3.5 Values and beliefs in practice

The NHS Constitution (Health Education England, 2021) provides a common set of NHS values, and by living these values staff can ensure the best possible care for patients: the key messages illustrate that everyone counts and that by working together we can improve the lives of our patients. The NHS values also make a commitment to quality care encompassing respect, dignity and compassion.

In addition, the NMC Code (NMC, 2018b) sets out the professional standards that patients and the public expect from health professionals on a daily basis. Local organisations have also developed their values in collaboration with patients, carers, staff and other stakeholders.

Our own values and beliefs are based on our own experiences, and our beliefs about mental illness can arise from several factors around us – our personal experiences, friends, family, the media and the community we live in. This could manifest itself in positive or negative attitudes, depending on our own experiences.

Nurses engage with a diverse group of people from all walks of life, with different beliefs and values around health that may conflict with our own beliefs and values. However, it is very important to consider and respect the cultural wishes, beliefs and experiences of patients when caring for them.

For example, some nurses may feel uncomfortable or scared to communicate with patients who appear to be hearing voices. Hearing voices can be triggered by several different factors – for example, bereavement, trauma, depression and psychosis – and not just in those who have a mental illness. Some of the voices can be very distressing for the patient and may involve voices from dead people. Others hear voices that they manage to live with daily and do not cause them any problems.

In this situation, it is important to speak to the patient and acknowledge their experience, and to find out what their coping strategies are or support them to develop their own. These could include distraction techniques, relaxation, listening to music or taking time to talk to the patient. By providing an empathic and compassionate approach you will not be challenging the patient's beliefs about the source of the voices, but supporting them in a patient-centred way.

ACTIVITY 3.2

How do you manage your own mental health?

What are your values, attitudes and beliefs about people with mental health conditions?

How might you approach someone who has a history of mental health issues in your working environment?

3.6 Person-centred and holistic care

Promoting holistic care is a value that underpins mental health care. Person-centred care highlights that patients are people first and are not defined by their condition, and that their needs should therefore be at the centre of care. It is important to recognise that all patients experience vulnerability when they are unwell and many patients with underlying mental health problems manage their condition very well without any major interventions. However, others may present with challenging or uncertain behaviour during a vulnerable time in their lives. Sometimes patients who are having a mental health crisis and are acutely unwell may act inappropriately – for example, they may expose themselves, use inappropriate language, be sexually disinhibited, insist on only you to facilitate their care, become upset if you are interacting with others and not with them, and so on. From time to time patients are unaware that they are even acting out of character and are very embarrassed once they have recovered. It is the responsibility of the nurse both to establish clear and appropriate boundaries and to support those who are vulnerable.

Person-centred care supports the notion that health care professionals work in collaboration with their patients to ensure that they receive the appropriate care for their needs. Person-centred care means focusing on a person's uniqueness and preferences. For example, person-centred care recognises dementia as only a diagnosis and that there is a person behind the diagnosis who should not be defined by their condition. They should still receive the same respect, privacy, dignity, rights and choices as everyone else.

3.7 Personal and professional boundaries

Maintaining boundaries and being professional is very important when engaging with patients and their families. Nurses are bound by a code of conduct, The Code (NMC, 2018b, p. 18), which states that, as a nurse, you must 'stay objective and have clear professional boundaries at all times with people in your care, their families and their carers'. Professional boundaries need to be built on trust and respect, and nurses need to consider their position of power.

Nurses have a legal responsibility not to share patient information and it is important that the patient knows that the information will be kept confidential. An empathic relationship encourages the sharing of personal feelings and views, allowing the patient to impart information that they might not ordinarily disclose. So the nurse needs to be aware of what they do with that information and respect the person's right to privacy. However, it is unacceptable for nurses to keep secrets for the patient, so nurses should make it clear to patients that on occasion they may have to breach confidentiality and tell other people involved in their care, particularly if there are serious concerns for the patient's own safety or public protection.

Nurses should be wary of excessive self-disclosure to patients and refrain from sharing details of their private lives. They should try to balance their conversations and remain respectful and courteous to the patient. For example, if a patient asks you a personal question you may need to think about where the conversation is going and whether the conversation may breach professional boundaries. You may also need to think about how you frame your response so that it maintains professional boundaries and doesn't upset the patient.

Therapeutic engagement with patients allows the nurse–patient relationship to become close; therefore nurses should maintain a professional alliance. The purpose of the therapeutic relationship is not to make friends or sexual partners, and if the relationship becomes too close and is at risk of crossing boundaries, someone else should be asked to take over the care of the patient.

ACTIVITY 3.3

Think about why someone with a mental health problem may not want to have information shared. How would you manage this dilemma, considering the principle of confidentiality and the professionalism required of being a nurse?

3.8 Patients transferred from a mental health setting

On occasion patients are transferred to a physical health care setting from a mental health unit for physical health care interventions and are escorted by members of staff from the mental health team. The patient may be detained under a section of the Mental Health Act 1983 and have restrictions outlined by Home Office regulations or be in a vulnerable condition that requires the patient to be closely monitored by regular mental health staff at all times. The safety of the patient, the staff and others is paramount; therefore, risk assessments will have been carried out prior to the transfer to ensure that the patient is appropriately supported while they receive care in a physical health care setting.

It may be a frightening experience meeting a patient for the first time when you are aware that they have been transferred from a mental health setting, particularly if they are being escorted by staff. Do not be afraid to ask for guidance from any escorting staff who are supporting the patient. They will have knowledge of the patient's vulnerabilities and if there are any flashpoints or triggers that may affect the patient's behaviour.

Building up therapeutic relationships with individuals who present with a variety of unfamiliar behaviours can be anxiety-provoking for the health care worker. What if the patient is hearing voices, presenting with paranoid behaviour, appears aggressive, is feeling suicidal, has self-harmed or is cognitively impaired? How do you know you are saying the right things, approaching the patient in the right way and not making things worse? Acknowledging the patient's feelings in a caring and compassionate way, by making eye contact and showing an interest as a person, is a good step for developing a therapeutic relationship. It is good practice to introduce yourself and to acknowledge the patient by their name; smiling and saying hello may seem obvious, but simple things can make a big difference. Ask how the patient would like to be called and communicate in a way that demonstrates a desire to listen and help. Random acts of kindness demonstrate that you genuinely care and value the patient – for example, finding time to talk to them and checking they are OK, not just when you are delivering interventions. It is also important to keep the patient involved and informed about the care they will receive, as this will reassure them that they are being listened to. Health care workers should never underestimate the positive therapeutic effect of being listened to (Ali, 2017).

Very often patients with a history of an acute mental health condition are placed in a side room away from others, sometimes through fear of putting them with other patients. In consequence some patients may feel ignored or rejected, so it is important that health care staff communicate with them periodically and do not rely on the escorting staff to carry out all of the interventions, so that the patient doesn't feel excluded.

On occasions a bed in a side ward may be justified if the patient poses a very high risk and is being supported by more than one escort, to preserve their dignity and to maintain safety.

ACTIVITY 3.4

John was admitted to a cardiac ward from home following an emergency call to 999 complaining of chest pain. He has a history of schizophrenia, which is currently stable. Suddenly, he politely refuses to take the medication that is vital for his physical health recovery.

Can you identify why John might have decided he does not want to take the medicine any more? How can you help him to understand his current physical illness? You may want to revisit sections above to assist you in answering, as there are many possible reasons.

3.9 **Challenging behaviour**

Challenging behaviour can be defined as any non-verbal, verbal or physical behaviour presented by a person that makes it problematic to deliver the appropriate care in a safe manner.

On occasion a patient may exhibit or experience challenging behaviour that impedes their physical health care. It may take many forms, such as patients being uncooperative, confused, argumentative, angry, aggressive or manipulative, refusing to have treatment or showing extreme emotional reactions. There may be a rational explanation for this behaviour, and by using active listening skills the situation may be resolved. However, on occasions nurses may require further support from mental health services to carry out their physical health care interventions. It is therefore important to manage the situation well by involving local mental health teams if necessary to carry out a mental health assessment and to provide further support. If the patient has been transferred from a local mental health service, it is advisable to contact the key practitioners as soon as difficulties arise.

Several mental health organisations have implemented an evidence-based model called Safewards. This model of care was designed to improve staff–patient working relationships to reduce 'conflict' and the need for containment. It is based on ten interventions that are mainly utilised in mental health inpatient settings, but several of the intervention techniques are transferable to more general physical health care settings (Safewards, 2020):

1. clear mutual expectations
2. soft words
3. talk down
4. positive words
5. bad news mitigation
6. know each other
7. mutual help meeting
8. calm down methods
9. reassurance
10. discharge messages.

Soft words: When a patient is acutely unwell, they can be difficult to manage, so think about the soft words you can use to demonstrate empathy, genuineness and warmth, and give attention to what they are saying.

Talk down: It is important to think about how you react to a crisis and about your own behaviour and how it may affect the patient. It is helpful to act in a calm and confident manner, with an open posture, demonstrating good eye contact but avoiding any confrontation. Try not to show any fear, anger or irritation, show no reaction to abusive language and remember that their behaviour is not personal. You may be required to move them away from others and into a safe environment. Maintain a physical distance, clarify what they are concerned about and offer to help them. Be congruent in your approach and use a concerned and interested tone of voice. You should demonstrate active listening skills by acknowledging the patient's feelings and discussing how the situation can be resolved.

Bad news mitigation: Be aware that on occasions you may have to give bad news, which may cause anger and upset. Staff–patient interaction can also be a trigger, particularly if you are saying 'no' to a patient's request. Bad news could relate to a variety of scenarios, such as their physical health condition, something that has happened at home or not being able to go home. By developing a therapeutic relationship with the patient and showing you are open and receptive to their concerns, you can enhance a collaborative patient–staff approach and encourage a dialogue of support. Patients may struggle to absorb the information and you may need to involve other members of the mental health multidisciplinary team to discuss strategies of how the news is conveyed or shared in the best interests of the patient.

Knowing each other: Opening communication channels and sharing common interests is a valuable way of developing a therapeutic relationship. In turn this can divert the person's attention away from their illness to talk about things that they are generally interested in. Some patients show subtle clues that their behaviour is about to change from their normal presentation. These may include tone of voice, restlessness, agitation, aggressive responses or other known indicators. A quick and effective response may be to give PRN medication, but there may be simpler interventions that have the same effect, such as taking time to talk to the patient about common interests or enjoying a cup of tea together. Conversation starters might include:

Nurse: *'What would be your dream holiday?'*

Nurse: *'What is your favourite food?'*

Nurse: *'What sort of music do you like?'*

ACTIVITY 3.5

Familiarise yourself with the Safewards website: www.safewards.net

How might the Safewards model help you to care for individuals with mental health conditions who require physical health care interventions?

What transferable skills and techniques could be implemented in your working environment to support all patients?

3.9.1 Conflict

Conflict can arise in any area in health care, between colleagues, managers, patients or their relatives and carers. Conflict is not necessarily about physical violence; it can be verbal conflict and disagreements in opinions, values, beliefs or actions, which can lead to avoidant behaviours and complaints within health care. It can be a disagreement between two or more people.

Individuals with mental health problems are sometimes thought of as violent because of portrayals in the media over recent years. However, a person experiencing a physical illness and, for example, an increase in pain can become agitated and irritable, contributing to conflict between them and the nurses caring for them. Likewise, someone with a physical health issue such as life-changing surgery, perhaps breast cancer resulting in a mastectomy, can appear irritable or angry after the operation. These could be signs of undiagnosed depression or signs of the grieving process from losing a part of their body, causing psychological distress. As a health care professional it is imperative that you can recognise signs of escalating conflict and not contribute to it.

Signs of conflict include:
- increase in tone, pitch and/or rate of speech
- tense, angry facial expression
- prolonged eye contact
- non-communication or withdrawal
- overarousal, including increased breathing and heart rate, muscle twitching
- verbal threats or gestures.

There are approaches and skills that you can use to de-escalate. Use a non-threatening, calming approach, taking care over your behaviour, posture and the tone and pitch of your voice, and being mindful of your proxemics. Promoting a mirroring approach, verbally by rephrasing the words used by the person and physically by remaining calm and in control, should result in the other person mimicking your behaviours and the conflict being minimised. Another approach is to structure the communication using a series of linked skills, which can be memorised using the acronym LEAPS:
- **L** – Listen
- **E** – Empathise
- **A** – Ask what the issue is
- **P** – Paraphrase what you have heard the person say to acknowledge understanding of their issues
- **S** – Summarise.

Remember that conflict is not an element of mental illness. Anybody can become angry or agitated as a result of their physical health problems. However, someone who is psychologically distressed may be more prone to becoming angry, upset or hostile. It is important here to use effective communication skills, while considering whether factors such as diagnostic overshadowing are affecting your ability to support the patient in your care.

At all times you need to be aware of your knowledge, skills and experience in dealing with these situations. Not all staff (including the most experienced) will be able to deal with all situations. You need to be aware of your own strengths but also your limitations and this may necessitate you asking for help. A good mantra is to know your limitations and always look after your own safety. Asking for help is not a weakness.

ACTIVITY 3.6

A 73-year-old woman has been recently diagnosed with dementia and has been admitted with severe abdominal pain.

What issues or challenges might you perceive in caring for this patient?

How might you approach her?

How could you involve the family/carers?

What steps might you take to ensure that the patient receives the care she needs?

CHAPTER SUMMARY

Key points to take away from *Chapter 3*:
- ☑ Effective communication is crucial in supporting someone with mental health problems.
- ☑ Be aware of the core conditions, knowledge and skills to support those in your care.
- ☑ Be self-aware and consider your values, personal and professional behaviour, when engaging with individuals with mental health problems.
- ☑ Recognise conflict and challenging behaviours and respond appropriately within your scope of practice.

Questions

Question 3.1   What are the key principles when communicating and relating to someone experiencing mental health problems? (*Learning outcome 3.1*)

Question 3.2   Discuss the core conditions required to support individuals with mental health problems. (*Learning outcome 3.2*)

Question 3.3   Describe the personal and professional behaviours needed in working with a person with mental health problems. (*Learning outcome 3.3*)

Question 3.4   Discuss the skills used in managing challenging behaviour (behaviours that challenge), including those where conflict may occur. (*Learning outcome 3.4*)

FURTHER READING

Health Education England (2021) *The NHS Constitutional Values Hub*. Available at: www.hee.nhs.uk/about/our-values/nhs-constitutional-values-hub-0 (accessed 23 June 2021).

Norman, K. (ed.) (2019) *Communication Skills: for nursing and healthcare students*. Lantern Publishing.

Nursing and Midwifery Council (2018) *The Code: professional standards of practice and behaviour for nurses, midwives and nursing associates*. Available at: www.nmc.org.uk/globalassets/sitedocuments/nmc-publications/nmc-code.pdf (accessed 23 June 2021).

Rogers, C.R. (1951) *Client Centred Therapy: its current practice, implications and theory*. Constable.

Safewards (2021) *Resources for Safewards Implementation*. Available at: www.safewards.net (accessed 23 June 2021).

Chapter 4

Nursing and caring for individuals with mental health problems

Elizabeth Burns, Emma Street, Shelly Allen and Lisa Bluff

LEARNING OUTCOMES

By the end of this chapter you should be able to:

4.1 Understand the different types of mental health difficulties

4.2 Understand the impact that mental health difficulties can have on individuals

4.3 Understand the different treatments and interventions.

4.1 Introduction

This chapter aims to provide an overview of mental health difficulties and how they are experienced. It will highlight some of the key interventions, with the intention of enabling you to have a fundamental knowledge of what to look for when working with people who access health services. Knowing what to look for is only one part of the role of any nurse; knowing what to do is another. Various interventions are introduced in this chapter, but from the outset, a nurse should only work within their range of understanding and confidence. We advocate that, if you are uncertain, you should ask a more experienced colleague or mental health practitioner.

Over recent years training packages have been developed around mental health first aid, and all registered nurses are expected to be able to administer basic mental health first aid (NMC, 2018a). Although this book does not directly address this as a bespoke theme, much of the basic understanding and evidence is addressed in the text. The knowledge of mental health first aid as provided in training packages, we believe, is only part of what all nurses require to both understand and intervene in when patients experience mental health problems. This book takes the knowledge and understanding further, and this will help you in determining how best to intervene, whether this is by providing therapeutic interventions yourself or identifying the need to involve other health care professionals to support the person.

As will become apparent throughout this chapter, we are all susceptible to mental health difficulties and some of the descriptions that follow may feel very familiar. Having a mental health difficulty does not equate to requiring intervention, because mental health exists on a continuum that we all travel in one direction or the other throughout our lives (see *Section 1.2.2*). It is the impact of the mental health difficulty that dictates whether we require therapeutic intervention and treatment, and being able to distinguish this is important in order to support the delivery of the right care at the right time by a thoughtful and skilled health care professional.

The NHS has further information and advice about the mental health difficulties discussed in this chapter – see www.nhs.uk/mental-health/conditions and www.nhs.uk/mental-health/feelings-symptoms-behaviours.

4.2 **Anxiety**

Anxiety disorders comprise several specific mental health conditions: generalised anxiety disorder, social anxiety disorder, post-traumatic stress disorder, panic disorder, obsessive–compulsive disorder and body dysmorphic disorder (NICE, 2014b). This section will focus on the signs and symptoms of generalised anxiety disorder, social anxiety disorder and panic disorder, and the impact on the life of an individual.

One in four adults will experience a mental health condition in any given year (NICE, 2019b). The 2014 Adult Psychiatric Morbidity Survey found that 19.7% of adults in England presented with symptoms of anxiety or depression, an increase of 15% in comparison to the previous year's survey (McManus *et al.*, 2016). Furthermore, the survey highlights that a third of self-identified sufferers did not have a formal diagnosis. It is therefore very likely that, as a health care student or practitioner, you will meet an individual with anxiety symptoms.

Anxiety is a feeling of unease, such as worry or fear, that can be mild or severe. It is a common human experience. For example, if you are having a job interview or delivering a presentation to a large audience, feeling anxious is completely normal and may even enhance performance. However, for some people anxiety can be constant and overwhelming and can affect their life significantly. The causes and symptoms of anxiety can be wide-ranging. For some it may be related to a particular trigger, such as social situations (NICE, 2013b). Others may experience more generalised symptoms, where they cannot identify a particular trigger and will describe feeling constantly anxious (NICE, 2011b).

Physical symptoms can include:
- dizziness
- tiredness
- dry mouth
- nausea

- headaches
- excessive sweating
- palpitations
- shaking or trembling
- muscle or stomach aches
- shortness of breath
- pins and needles
- insomnia.

These symptoms may be mistake
patients and health professionals.
experience psychological sympto
feeling irritable, having difficulty (
(NICE, 2014b).

Just as the symptoms can be varie
person's life. Symptoms can be mi
find ways to minimise the impact
anxiety – for example, shopping d

However, for some, anxiety can be extremely debilitating and its impact can be significant in terms of employment, self-esteem, mood, physical health, finances and relationships. Just as the impact can be debilitating for the individual, it can also affect the lives of their families and others close to them.

There are different treatments available to help people with anxiety. It is important to note, however, that one size does not fit all. When considering treatment options, a personalised approach should be used and decisions about treatments should be made collaboratively by the health care team and the individual (NICE, 2011b). NICE (2014b) recommends psychological therapies such as CBT for all patients with anxiety. However, it also provides advice about the use of different types of medication in conjunction with psychological therapies, where these are indicated, based on individual need. The increased focus on personalisation in health care has led to the recognition that a person's health is determined by a range of social, environmental and economic factors too and that there are wider non-clinical services within communities that can provide support to individuals to enable them to take greater control of their own health and emotional wellbeing (King's Fund, 2020). Social prescribing initiatives have demonstrated that they can be effective methods of support for individuals with anxiety disorder (NHS England and NHS Improvement, 2019). There are many examples of social prescribing and these vary across different locations, but can include activities such as healthy eating groups, exercise/sports groups and volunteering.

4.3 Obsessive–compulsi

Obsessive–compulsive disorder
which a person has recurren[+]
that they feel the urge to
2020). In the UK, appro
a diagnosis of OCD
health diagnose[']
it is highly lik[']
greater (M
across[i]

Th[']

ACTIVITY 4.1

As we have said, anxiety can happen to anyone. Think back to a time when you felt anxious – for example, your university/job interview. How did you feel? What do you think would have helped?

...sorder

...CD) is a common and long-lasting disorder in
...noughts (obsessions) and/or behaviours (compulsions)
...peat over and over (National Institute of Mental Health,
...mately 1–3% of adults and around 0.25% of children have
...NICE, 2018a). It is also worth noting that, as with other mental
...people experiencing symptoms fear stigmatisation and therefore
...y that the true number of people experiencing OCD symptoms is
...Manus *et al.*, 2016). It is therefore also highly likely that you will come
...dividuals within practice with OCD.

...e ways in which OCD can present can be wide-ranging in terms of symptoms,
severity and the impact that it has on an individual's life. Some people describe
experiencing repeated thoughts, urges or mental images that cause feelings of
anxiety. These are known as *obsessions*. Examples of these include fear of germs,
the need for things to be in a perfect order, unwanted repetitive and intrusive
thoughts that cause distress, and aggressive thoughts towards others or self
(NICE, 2018a).

Other people experience what are known as *compulsions*. These are repetitive
behaviours that a person feels the urge to do as a response to an obsessive thought,
for example excessive cleaning, ordering things in a certain way or repeatedly
checking that the iron is switched off. Some of these thoughts, feelings and
behaviours will be familiar to many of us; however, the difference is the distress
and the impact that they can cause. A person with OCD is likely to be unable to
control the thoughts or behaviours. They will not get pleasure from performing the
behaviour, but will experience temporary relief from the anxiety that the thoughts
cause, and the impact on their lives will be significant (National Institute of Mental
Health, 2020). For some, the need to repeatedly check that appliances are switched
off, for example, may lead to problems in the workplace because they are constantly
late; or it could be that the nature of the intrusive thoughts is so distressing that they
are experiencing thoughts of self-harm or suicide.

If not treated, OCD usually persists. Depending on the individual and the severity
of symptoms there is a range of treatment options. These may include individual
or group psychological treatments such as CBT (including exposure and response
prevention therapy) and, where appropriate, medication. Involving the person's
family/carers is a helpful part of any psychosocial intervention as this can add an
extra layer of support to the individual between therapy sessions (NICE, 2005).

4.4 Post-traumatic stress disorder

Post-traumatic stress disorder (PTSD) is classed as an anxiety disorder caused by an
exceptionally threatening or frightening event or situation. It is usually a delayed or
protracted response (but it can occur immediately) to an event/situation that is likely
to cause distress to almost anyone.

In the UK, it is estimated that around 3% of adults will experience PTSD (McManus *et al.*, 2016) and that one in three people who experiences a traumatic event will be affected by PTSD (Greenberg, Brooks and Dunn, 2015). There is no agreed definition as to what a traumatic event/situation is, but examples include rare but severe events such as combat or natural disasters. However, PTSD can also be related to many other stress-inducing events, such as car accidents, traumatic pregnancies and births, prolonged bullying, neglect, abuse, bereavement or a significant change in health status (see www.ptsduk.org/what-is-ptsd). The lack of clarity regarding what is considered a traumatic event and the differing theories in relation to why some people experience PTSD and some do not (e.g. that childhood adversity and development, personality traits, etc. play a role) make diagnosis and consequently treatment complex.

As with other diagnoses, the symptoms and impact of PTSD can be varied. Common symptoms include:

- **Re-experiencing** – this can be in the form of flashbacks, nightmares, repetitive distressing images, or thoughts that try to make sense of what has happened.
- **Avoidance** – this may be in relation to people or places that remind the person of the trauma.
- **Distraction** – sometimes people will invest lots of time in hobbies, work, etc. to avoid thinking about the trauma.
- **Emotional numbing** – sometimes feelings can be so overwhelming that a person deals with them by trying to not feel at all. This can lead to social isolation and withdrawal.
- **Hyperarousal** – sometimes people will describe feeling constantly anxious and unable to relax. This can present as irritability, anger, and difficulties sleeping and concentrating.
- **Dissociation** – a person might feel disconnected or detached from themselves or from the world around them.
- **Negative self-perception** – feeling defeated or worthless.

Some people experience other problems alongside PTSD, such as depression, anxiety, substance misuse and physical symptoms such as headaches, dizziness and chest pains (NICE, 2018b).

As discussed above, PTSD can be varied in terms of severity and impact. For some, it can have an impact on relationships, work, etc. and it is therefore important that people have access to appropriate treatments. As with other mental health diagnoses, depending on the individual and the severity of symptoms there is a range of treatment options. These can include psychological therapies such as trauma-focused CBT or eye movement desensitisation and reprocessing (EMDR), and/or medication. Please note that EMDR is a highly specialised therapy practised by accredited CBT therapists, but it is becoming a more widely used therapy for people experiencing trauma. Most nurses will probably only need to be aware of this specialist treatment, as it is a bespoke skill that requires several layers of further training.

In all cases, it is important that the individual needs of the patient are assessed (NICE, 2018b).

4.5 **Depression**

Depression is a common mental health problem that causes people to experience low mood, loss of interest or pleasure, feelings of guilt or low self-worth, disturbed sleep or appetite, low energy and poor concentration (Mental Health Foundation, 2018; NICE, 2009). As discussed earlier in this chapter, the 2014 Adult Psychiatric Morbidity Survey found that 19.7% of adults in England presented with symptoms of anxiety or depression (McManus *et al.*, 2016).

The causes of depression are complex and can be related to biological, psychological and/or social factors (Fallon, 2019). For some, a significant adverse event such as bereavement, relationship breakdown or loss of a job can trigger symptoms of depression. Women are almost twice as likely to suffer from depression as men, and individuals with long-term conditions such as diabetes or heart disease are at increased risk of developing symptoms of depression. Therefore, when working with all individuals, we should be alert to this and provide appropriate levels of support. As a health care professional within any field of practice, it is highly likely that you will work with patients with a diagnosis of depression or depressive symptoms. Recognising symptoms and being able to support individuals is therefore of paramount importance.

The ways in which depression can present can be wide-ranging in terms of symptoms, severity and the impact that it has on an individual's life. For some it can lead to difficulties at home, at work and in family life. Some will avoid contact with friends and family and stop engaging in hobbies or other interests. What is clear is that there is still a considerable amount of stigma associated with depression, with some perceiving it as a sign of weakness. When we consider this with the clear links between depression and self-harming and suicidal thoughts and behaviours (Fallon, 2019), it is clear that we all have a responsibility to ensure that individuals receive appropriate support and treatment depending on their needs (NICE, 2011b).

Many people who experience mild depression will recover without the need for any treatment (Fallon, 2019) and therefore the role of health care professionals may be just supportive in nature, engaging in a non-judgemental relationship that is based on openness and facilitating conversations that are based on hope and optimism (NICE, 2009). For others, the addition of low-intensity psychological therapies such as CBT either through self-help strategies or group approaches may be of benefit. Where symptoms persist, or depression is assessed to be moderate to severe, medication may be required in addition to more intensive psychological therapies. However, as with all diagnoses and treatments, a person-centred approach is needed to ensure that each person is offered interventions that are reflective of the evidence base and their individual needs.

ACTIVITY 4.2

Many of us have experienced a situation that has affected our mood or have had someone in our family or friendship group who has felt sad or low in mood. Please think back to what this looked like. What impact did this have on your/your family member's/ friend's life? What do you think would have helped?

4.6 Bipolar disorder

The NHS describes bipolar disorder as a mental health problem that affects a person's mood. People who experience this difficulty will have mood swings that range from feeling very depressed to very elated. When they feel high in mood they may appear to be overactive and have difficulty sleeping. They often believe that they have special abilities and can sometimes spend large amounts of money in a short space of time. When they feel low they will often lose interest in things and may have thoughts about wanting to end their life. There are three main types of bipolar disorder, so it is important that people are assessed by a mental health professional to try to establish which one they have:

- **bipolar I** – if a person has experienced at least one episode of mania that lasted longer than a week
- **bipolar II** – if a person has experienced at least one episode of severe depression and hypomania
- **cyclothymia** – if a person has experienced both hypomanic and depressive moods over the course of 2 years or more and their symptoms are not severe enough to meet the criteria for bipolar I or II.

About one in 50 people will develop bipolar disorder at some point in their life and it usually starts between the ages of 15 and 25, but very rarely after the age of 50 (NICE, 2020a). There are several effective treatments, and medications are usually the first treatment option that people will use. These medications are broadly divided into those that keep someone's mood stable and those that treat a depressive or manic episode.

The most common mood stabiliser for the treatment of bipolar disorder is lithium. This medication is very effective (Butler *et al.*, 2018), but it needs to be initiated by a psychiatrist as it is difficult to get the level of lithium right. If the level is too low then it will not be effective; on the other hand, if it is too high then there is a danger that it can cause physical complications such as kidney damage. To monitor this, regular blood tests are taken, but lithium levels are very sensitive to the amount of water in the body (NICE, 2020a). Therefore, if a patient taking lithium for a pre-existing diagnosis of bipolar disorder is admitted for a physical health concern, it is imperative that lithium blood levels are recorded and signs of dehydration closely monitored.

Other mood stabilisers can be used, and these are often anti-epileptic drugs such as carbamazepine and lamotrigine. Sodium valproate should never be prescribed to women of childbearing age, because of the high risk of birth defects and reduction in IQ of babies born to women who take the drug when pregnant (NICE, 2020a).

Psychological therapies can be very beneficial during either a depressive or manic episode (Oud *et al.*, 2016). CBT can help people to recover from depressive states and to identify when their mood might be changing. People will usually have 16–20 sessions, which usually take about three to four months to complete.

4.7 **Psychosis**

The term psychosis is used to describe when people lose touch with reality. Sometimes people hear or see things that others cannot see (*hallucinations*), or they experience *delusions* where they believe things that are not true. Psychosis can be a symptom of other mental health difficulties, such as schizophrenia, bipolar disorder or depression. However, people can also experience psychosis when they have a severe infection (*delirium*), severe stress and anxiety or lack of sleep. Some people experience psychosis after they take recreational drugs such as cannabis and LSD (Vallersnes *et al.*, 2016). There are also medical conditions that can trigger a psychotic episode, such as HIV and AIDS, Alzheimer's disease, Parkinson's disease, hypoglycaemia, lupus and multiple sclerosis.

When caring for someone with psychosis it is important to perform a comprehensive physical examination first to ensure that there is no underlying physical cause before continuing to a mental health assessment. This is commonly completed by the admitting doctor, although nurses who are trained in such areas, for example advanced clinical practitioners, may undertake the examination and 'clerking in' of the person.

If the psychosis is due to a mental health difficulty, then clients are usually treated with an antipsychotic medication that works by blocking the effect of dopamine on the brain. It is thought that a disruption in how this neurotransmitter relays information may play an important part in the development of psychosis. CBT is also beneficial for people who experience psychosis as part of their mental health difficulty, as it can help them understand and cope with their auditory hallucinations. It has been recommended by NICE (2014c) for people who have their first episode of psychosis, as along with medication it can delay the onset of future episodes and reduce the impact of current ones.

4.8 **Schizophrenia**

Schizophrenia is a mental health problem that affects the way in which people think, feel and behave. Many people believe that schizophrenia means someone has a 'split personality', but this is not the case. Schizophrenia is a type of psychosis that affects approximately one in every 100 people and usually starts in young adulthood (NICE, 2014c). Both men and women are equally liable to develop it. The symptoms of schizophrenia are usually divided into positive and negative symptoms. *Positive symptoms* are extra things that people feel, sense or think, which can include hearing voices, having beliefs about the world that other people do not have (delusions) and disorganised thinking, where the person talks very quickly and it is often hard to keep track of their meaning. When people hear voices, these are real to the person; the voices often have a distinct accent, gender and age and they seem to come from outside, so people will often turn in their direction. *Negative symptoms* are similar to depression, as people often lack motivation and experience a change in sleep patterns and social withdrawal.

There are effective treatments that enable people to recover and manage their illness. Once diagnosed, a combination of antipsychotic medication and CBT is often prescribed. There are many different types of antipsychotic and they are very effective in helping people manage both the negative and positive symptoms (Leucht *et al.*, 2013). CBT has also been shown to be helpful in managing the effects of positive symptoms (Turner *et al.*, 2014). In addition, social skills training, which is a type of psychotherapy in which people learn to become more socially competent, is very effective for individuals who struggle with their negative symptoms (Almerie *et al.*, 2015).

4.9 **Self-harm**

The NICE (2013a) quality standard refers to self-harm as any act of self-poisoning or self-injury, regardless of motivation, and it commonly includes actions such as overdosing and cutting. Actions such as accidental harm to oneself, problems with eating and excessive consumption of alcohol or recreational drugs are excluded from this definition of self-harm. In terms of offering an operational definition, NICE has captured what would typically be considered to constitute self-harm. However, the acts excluded from this definition may also be a form of self-harm, and if a strict definition is used it may mean that people who would benefit from therapeutic intervention and signposting to relevant help are missed. An example of this is someone who repeatedly attends the A&E department following fights. They may be sensitively cared for and their physical injuries addressed, thereby leading to a good outcome in this respect. However, if such a pattern is noticed and they are gently encouraged to explore why they find themselves in this situation, it may be that the reasons are less about being angry with others and relate more to how they feel about themselves.

Turp (2002) urges a focus not on the physical manifestation of harm but on the states of mind that underlie it. For non-mental health professionals this may seem a daunting prospect, but people who have used services following self-harm repeatedly say that one of the most helpful aspects was being treated with compassion and understanding. This was also reported by Saunders *et al.* (2012), who found that the attitudes and knowledge of clinical staff in relation to self-harm are likely to influence clinical practice and the experiences and outcomes for people using services.

Conversely, poor attitude and knowledge can lead to poor outcomes. Experts by experience are people who have had experience of services as a user or a carer in the past five years, whose observations and experiences are used to shape services (CQC, 2020). They share experiences of care following self-harm that has not just been found wanting but that has also been damaging. Contemporary health care practice has no place for such experiences, and it is therefore of paramount importance that all health care professionals learn how to work effectively with people who engage with services following self-harm.

This need prompted NICE (2013a) to state explicitly that people who attend services following self-harm must be cared for compassionately and with dignity. Given that training health care professionals leads to consistent improvements in attitude and knowledge regarding self-harm and that general hospital is typically the most common place that people attend following this, it is crucial that staff are afforded opportunities to develop the necessary knowledge and skills to support people to ensure a compassionate and dignified response.

4.10 Suicidal feelings

A House of Commons briefing paper (Mackley, 2019) drew on the then latest Office for National Statistics report (ONS, 2019) that there were 6,507 recorded suicides in the UK in 2018, that this was an increase on preceding years and was the highest rate since 2002. Suicidal feelings are not rare; they fall on a continuum, from fleeting and infrequent to pervasive, intrusive and leading to action. The expression of suicidal feelings by people who use services can be anxiety-provoking for health care professionals and there may be a tendency to try to avoid such issues. However, evidence indicates that feeling safe enough to talk about them can be protective, and organisations such as Samaritans have demonstrated this repeatedly. Cole-King *et al.* (2013) provide helpful prompts aimed at the clarification of suicidal thoughts and intent, which can help health care professionals when exploring this with people who engage with services.

Feeling confident and competent enough to do this is crucial in 'making every contact count' (PHE, 2018a), given that health care professionals are ideally placed to support people who are experiencing suicidal feelings, particularly when the link with chronic physical illness is considered. This is supported by Cole-King *et al.* (2013), who state that it is the quality of the therapeutic relationship that makes disclosure of suicidal thoughts possible and that asking about suicidal thoughts is the first step in reducing the risk.

NICE (2013a) states that people who self-harm have a 50 to 100 times higher likelihood of dying by suicide in the 12-month period after an episode than people who do not self-harm. The overlap between self-harm and suicide is complicated and should be explored sufficiently to enable a thoughtful, useful response. This is in keeping with Cole-King *et al.* (2013), who state that all suicidal thoughts require a compassionate, proportionate and timely response. For health professionals, this requires refraining from over-controlling strategies, which may increase suicide risk, and avoiding the temptation not to take the threat seriously enough and thereby failing to ensure adequate care and support. Work by authors such as Cole-King *et al.* (2013), who provide guidance on how to assess suicide risk and suggest strategies to put in place to minimise this risk, offers useful resources to draw on.

It is also important to note that suicidal thoughts are influenced by demographics and the life course. In a systematic review of suicidal behaviour in older adults, Fung and Chan (2011) found that women were more likely to engage in repeated attempts, whereas men were more likely to engage in what were referred to as severe attempts. The highest rate of suicide was found to be in men over 75, with widowed men being particularly at risk. Serious physical illness in men was notable, and wishing to die was strongly associated with depression. Contact with doctors was frequent up to the last three months before suicide and then declined. In contrast, the lowest suicide rates have been recorded in males aged 10 to 24 years. However, in 2018 this rate increased by 25% compared with figures for the same group in 2017 (ONS, 2019). In the same report it is stated that the suicide rate among females aged 10 to 24 also increased to its highest recorded level since 1981.

When acting on suicidal feelings, young people may be less likely to leave a suicide note or spend a long time planning and instead be impulsive. This differs from what is typically understood to indicate high risk and these differences in relation to suicidality across demographics must be understood and taken into account. In doing this, a compassionate stance as advocated by Cole-King *et al.* (2013) must form part of all health care professionals' clinical practice and can be used in conjunction with guidance on undertaking a comprehensive assessment of suicidal feelings.

4.11 Eating disorders

Everybody has a relationship with food. Eating is a big part of life for many, from both a physiological perspective and an emotional perspective. Eating with families and friends can be a rich social activity with enormous psychological benefits, but an individual's relationship with food can develop into a negative coping mechanism to handle emotional distress. Then the relationship is based solely on the notion of controlling weight. This may be in response to a range of triggers, such as neurochemical changes, genetics, lack of confidence, low self-esteem, bullying or other difficulties.

Preoccupation with food is a big part of an individual's eating disorder, but the issues are much broader and more complex for most. However, the preoccupation with food can sometimes be the only outward sign that the individual is in emotional distress (Wright and McKeown, 2018).

Eating disorders can be difficult to diagnose, and diagnosis is often made on the basis of the person's history and clinical features, and supported, where possible, by corroboration from a relative or friend. There is a misperception that eating disorders only affect women and girls – this is not true. Eating disorders are more prevalent in females (Fallon, 2019), but they can occur in anyone of any age, gender or ethnic background (Wright and McKeown, 2018). Some individuals will present with non-specific symptoms, such as fatigue, dizziness or lack of energy, or physical complications associated with starvation, purging and vomiting (NICE, 2019a).

There are three main types of eating disorder: anorexia nervosa, bulimia nervosa and binge eating disorder.

Individuals with a diagnosis of *anorexia nervosa*, in addition to the above symptoms, will usually present as underweight (at least 15% below that expected for the person) and will avoid foods that they believe are fattening. They may also engage in what are known as compensatory behaviours, such as self-induced vomiting and/or laxative use, excessive exercise and the use of appetite suppressants or diuretics. Psychological features may include body image distortion and denial that there is a problem.

Individuals with *bulimia nervosa* will usually engage in recurrent episodes of binge eating, in addition to compensatory behaviours. They may experience anxiety and mood disturbances, and feel persistently preoccupied with thoughts of food and feelings of guilt and shame about their behaviour.

Although the symptoms of bulimia and binge eating disorder overlap in terms of binge eating, compensatory behaviours and high levels of distress and mood disturbance, *binge eating disorder* is also associated with feeling a loss of control over how much is being eaten. Additionally (although not always), people with this disorder are more likely to be obese or overweight.

In terms of interventions and treatments, a personalised approach is needed, with evidence supporting the use of psychological therapies, dietary counselling and medication as appropriate (NICE, 2020c).

4.12 Mental health difficulties in pregnancy and beyond

Any mental health problem that occurs between conception and up to one year after the child's birth comes under the heading of a perinatal mental health difficulty. This is because there are differences in the way that it can be experienced and treated when pregnancy is involved.

There is a misconception that when a woman is pregnant, she does not feel depressed or anxious. However, this is not necessarily the case, and it is estimated that around 12% of pregnant women experience depression at some point in the antenatal period and 13% experience anxiety. Many experience both, and this rises to 15–20% in the first year after birth (NICE, 2014a). Some women who experience mental illness in the perinatal period have no history of mental health problems; some who do have such a history feel that their mental health deteriorates at this time. This could be due to physical, social and psychological changes or changing medication (Hogg, 2013).

ACTIVITY 4.3	

Think about all the changes that happen to a woman when she is pregnant. Try to list all the things under three headings:
1. Physical
2. Psychological
3. Social

Suicide is the second most common cause of women's death while pregnant and the leading cause of maternal death during the first year after pregnancy (Knight *et al.*, 2019). The ways in which women take their own life during this period are different from those seen in the general female population. Women in the perinatal period are more likely to take their life by violent means and very suddenly, and this leaves very little time for people or services to intervene.

Women who report any of the following symptoms need **urgent** referral to a specialist perinatal mental health team – it may be necessary to contact 999 if there is immediate risk of harm:

- new thoughts of violent self-harm
- sudden onset or rapidly worsening mental symptoms
- persistent feelings of estrangement from their baby.

4.12.1 Antenatal anxiety and depression

During pregnancy and after having a baby it is normal to feel worried and anxious. However, sometimes this worry can increase to the point that it affects how a person lives their life and their feelings towards their pregnancy and baby. Often anxiety and depression during the perinatal period are attributed to hormones, or their importance is minimised. This can make it difficult for women to express how they feel. Anxiety during pregnancy may be more common than depression (Ross and McLean, 2006) and, if left untreated, can have long-lasting effects on both mother and infant. Mothers may find it difficult to bond with their baby and avoid interacting with their infant because of intrusive thoughts or intense anxiety.

There is a solid evidence base for the use of CBT in treating perinatal anxiety (Wenzel and Kleiman, 2015). It can help people to develop an understanding of the thoughts, feelings and behaviours that relate to their anxiety, which in turn can have a positive effect on their ability to parent.

4.12.2 Postnatal anxiety and depression

Postnatal depression is the most widely researched of all the perinatal mental health difficulties. Symptoms of depression and anxiety have been found to emerge two to six weeks post delivery (RCPsych, 2015). Someone is more likely to develop postnatal depression and anxiety if they have experienced the following (Stewart *et al.*, 2003):

- previous depression or anxiety
- recent stressful events
- domestic abuse
- poor support from loved ones.

It is not only mothers who can experience postnatal depression; there is a growing body of evidence showing that fathers also experience it. It is thought that around 10% of new fathers have symptoms of depression or anxiety, but it is conceivable that the prevalence may be much higher (Paulson and Bazemore, 2010).

There is evidence to suggest that postpartum depression is associated with several negative infant and child outcomes, including poor cognitive functioning, insecure attachment and social maladjustment (Murray and Cooper, 2003). However, these effects can be mitigated with effective and timely treatment.

When working with a mother who you suspect of having postnatal depression or anxiety, it is important to check to see whether there is an underlying physical cause. An underactive thyroid, low levels of vitamin B12 and anaemia are common after childbirth and can mimic the signs of depression, whereas an overactive thyroid can present as if someone is anxious.

4.12.3 Postpartum psychosis

Postpartum psychosis (PPP) or puerperal psychosis is a rare but serious mental health problem that affects approximately one in every 1,000 women who have a baby (VanderKruik *et al.*, 2017). Unlike some other mental health problems, symptoms of PPP can develop within hours or days after giving birth and can include hallucinations, elated mood, confusion and depression (Heron *et al.*, 2008). If you think someone may have PPP it is important that you get specialist help quickly, as it is a **psychiatric emergency**. Any mother can develop PPP but women who have a family history or a diagnosis of bipolar disorder are at more risk (Di Florio, Smith and Jones, 2013).

Treatment usually consists of a combination of antipsychotic medication and a talking therapy such as CBT (NICE, 2014a). As PPP is such a serious mental health condition, women are often admitted to specialist psychiatric wards called mother and baby units (MBUs). These acute mental health units can care for both mother and baby, which is beneficial in maintaining and developing the bonding relationship. They usually only have 6–12 clients and the staff includes mental health professionals and nursery nurses. Following discharge, women are normally referred to the perinatal community psychiatric team for continued support.

4.13 Alcohol and drug use disorders

To develop a contemporary understanding of alcohol and drug use disorders, it is helpful first to identify popular types of psychoactive substance used in the UK and worldwide. In their original dictionary of alcohol and drug terminology, the World Health Organization (WHO, 1994) defines a psychoactive substance as any drug ingested or administered that 'changes the cognition and/or the affect of the user'. Psychoactive substances can broadly be categorised into three main types according to their intoxicating effects on the central nervous system:

- **stimulant drugs** (nicotine, cocaine, amphetamines, ecstasy, MDMA)
- **hallucinogens and dissociative drugs** (LSD, magic mushrooms, ketamine)
- **depressant drugs** (alcohol, opiates, benzodiazepines).

Cannabis, on the other hand, is a drug that has long been argued not to fit as neatly into one clear group, owing to its combined stimulant, hallucinogenic, dissociative and depressant effects (Ashton, 2001).

There are a number of different alcohol or drug use disorders, and these are generally defined in terms of severity (ranging from hazardous to harmful to dependent use) according to future risk posed or evidence of current harm (WHO, 2018a; WHO and United Nations Office on Drugs and Crime, 2020).

It is important to understand that alcohol and drug use disorders are classified separately from their legal status and that people experience difficulties along a continuum of harm. Although alcohol is a legal psychoactive drug, research suggests that it is the most harmful drug, with heroin and crack cocaine in second and third place (Nutt, King and Phillips, 2010). However, scientific attempts to rank the harmful effects of different drugs are not necessarily reflected in the public's perception of harm or national drug policy such as the Misuse of Drugs Act 1971 (Cheeta *et al.*, 2018).

Traditionally, psychoactive drugs have been derived from plants – examples include cocaine, heroin and cannabis (WHO and United Nations Office on Drugs and Crime, 2020) – but more recently, 'new psychoactive substances' (NPS) have emerged that can be described as synthetic drugs manufactured to mimic the effects of long-established recreational drugs (Tracy, Wood and Baumeister, 2017). Furthermore, and often under the radar, there have been increasing concerns about dependence and withdrawal problems associated with prescription or over-the-counter medicines such as benzodiazepines, Z-drugs (the sedatives zopiclone, zolpidem and zaleplon), opioid pain medicines, gabapentinoids and antidepressants (PHE, 2019b). The term 'alcohol and drug use disorders' should therefore be taken to include the difficulties people can experience because of illegal substances (controlled in the UK under the Misuse of Drugs Act 1971), legal drugs such as alcohol (controlled under the Licensing Act 2003), as well as prescribed drugs or over-the-counter medication (controlled under the Medicines Act 1968).

The prevalence of alcohol and drug use in England is outlined in the following statistics:

- One in four adults (25.7%) report drinking more than the lower risk guidelines of 14 units of alcohol each week (PHE, 2020b).
- In 2018/2019, there were 358,000 admissions to hospital where the main reason was alcohol consumption – 19% higher than in 2008/2009 (NHS Digital, 2020).
- One in five young adults (20.3%) aged 16–24 report taking an illicit drug in the past year, compared with almost one in ten adults (9.4%) aged 16–59 (NHS Digital, 2019).
- In 2018/2019, there were 18,053 hospital admissions due to poisoning from drug use – 16% higher than in 2012/2013 (NHS Digital, 2019).
- Deaths related to poisoning by drug use increased by 46% between 2008 and 2018 (NHS Digital, 2019).

The harmful effects of different substances can vary according to several different factors: the amount used, frequency of use, duration of use, route of administration as well as the context of use. There are physical, psychological and social harms (Nutt, King and Phillips, 2010; WHO, 2018a; WHO and United Nations Office on Drugs and Crime, 2020). Alcohol alone has been found to be a causal factor in over 200 medical conditions because of acute intoxication or regular use over time (PHE, 2019a). Co-occurring mental health issues are common, with 70% of drug service users and 86% of alcohol service users having an identifiable mental health problem (PHE, 2017). Hidden harms of alcohol and drug use have tragically only come to light following local enquiries (serious case reviews) into the death of, or serious injury to, children who have been neglected or abused, with parental alcohol or drug use being a feature in 47% of cases (PHE, 2018b).

Risk-based language is recommended when assessing a person's risk of harm from alcohol and/or drug use: the four typical classifications are low risk, hazardous, harmful and dependent use. When exploring the difficulties people may face in relation to alcohol or other drug use, language becomes important. To promote engagement and potential behaviour change, Miller and Rollnick (2012) describe the effectiveness of 'counselling with neutrality' – in other words, avoiding language that implies judgement, imposes or tries to influence choices or goals, or compounds stigma. Fundamentally, the high prevalence of co-occurring mental health conditions alongside alcohol or drug use means that in practice there are two key principles that should underpin interventions for alcohol and drug use disorders (PHE, 2017, p. 25):

■ It is everyone's job – co-occurring conditions are the norm rather than the exception, and commissioners and providers of mental health and alcohol and drug use services have a joint responsibility to work collaboratively to meet the needs of people with co-occurring conditions.

■ There is no wrong door – providers in alcohol and drug, mental health and other services have an open door policy for individuals with co-occurring conditions. Commissioning enables services to respond collaboratively, effectively and flexibly to presenting needs and to prevent exclusion, and services should offer compassionate and non-judgemental care that is centred on the person's needs and is accessible from every point of contact.

To do this, a first step is to be able to identify drug or alcohol use using a short 'risk identification tool' in routine practice (NICE, 2010; NICE, 2017). For example, ASSIST-Lite is a tool in widespread use in health and social care settings in the UK and it aims to support early identification of and intervention in alcohol and drug use disorders (PHE, 2020a).

Brief interventions should be offered in the form of a structured conversation such as 'very brief advice' using Ask, Advise, Act (less than five minutes) or 'brief advice' using the FRAMES approach (five to ten minutes) (PHE, 2020a). Brief interventions are based on the core principles of motivational interviewing (Miller and Rollnick, 2012), although the word 'brief' does not necessarily reflect the complexity of communication skill required of the practitioner (Miller and Rollnick, 2009). The COM-B model (Michie, van Stralen and West, 2011) can help us to understand the mechanism of action underpinning brief interventions. This model attends to 'motivation' as one integral aspect of behaviour change, alongside exploring a person's capability and opportunity to change. Although it remains popular, more awareness is needed among health and social care professionals of the limitations of using the Stages of Change model as the default behaviour change approach (West, 2005).

Beyond brief interventions, treatment for alcohol and drug use disorders can include several different options. According to the National Drug and Alcohol Treatment

Monitoring System for England (PHE, 2020c), these 'high level' interventions provided by specialist alcohol and drug treatment services can be subdefined as:

- pharmacological interventions
- psychosocial interventions
- recovery interventions.

Different approaches to pharmacological management of alcohol and drug use disorders include: assisted physical withdrawal; short- or long-term harm reduction; substitution; maintenance of abstinence; and the acute management of medical emergencies (Lingford-Hughes *et al.*, 2012). Although alcohol is a legal drug, as noted above it is perhaps the most harmful drug and the medical emergencies that can arise from alcohol withdrawal can be life-threatening or life-limiting. Vigilance is therefore needed during unplanned admissions to hospital for withdrawal seizures, delirium tremens and Wernicke's encephalopathy (NICE, 2011a).

In relation to psychosocial interventions, research suggests several options, including motivational interviewing, contingency management, family and social network interventions, cognitive and behaviour-based relapse prevention, 12-step work, and psychological or psychotherapy interventions for co-occurring mental health problems (PHE, 2020c).

Recovery support has largely developed from 'asset-based approaches' to wellbeing (PHE, 2015). These use the 'assets' – for example, peer support or mutual aid organisations – available to the person and they continue beyond what may be defined as a period of 'structured treatment'.

Overall, taking a social approach to the prevention and treatment of alcohol and drug use disorders requires action to reduce health inequalities, addressing the 'causes of the causes' or the social determinants of health (Marmot *et al.*, 2020). However, a careful balance is needed, since specialist medical interventions remain necessary, particularly in the context of assisted withdrawal, harm reduction or abstinence support, as well as the management of medical and/or mental health emergencies. To make every contact count, early intervention and treatment for people with co-occurring conditions need to be available at every contact point.

ACTIVITY 4.4

When completing a short risk identification tool to assess alcohol use, it is important to understand the unit content of popular alcoholic drinks. There are lots of unit calculators available online or you could use the following formula (1 UK Unit = 10 ml of pure alcohol):

Abv (%) x Volume (ml) ÷ 1000 = Units (rounded up to one decimal point)

Example: 12% wine, large glass (250 ml)

12 x 250 ÷ 1000 = 3 units

Large glass of 12% wine = 3 units	Bottle of 12% wine = 9 units
Double gin and tonic = 2 units	70 cl bottle of 40% spirits = 28 units
500 ml can of 4% lager = 2 units	1 litre of 7.5% cider = 7.5 units

4.14 **Personality disorders**

The NHS describes a person with a diagnosis of a personality disorder as someone who thinks, feels, behaves or relates to others differently from the average person. The ICD-11 Classification of Mental and Behavioural Disorders (WHO, 2019a) names ten specific personality disorders and the diagnostic criteria relevant to each. It is reasonable to suggest, however, that the use of personality disorder as a diagnosis is not without controversy.

In their systematic review of service user, clinician and carer perspectives of mental health diagnosis, Perkins *et al.* (2018) state that personality disorder was regarded as having all the drawbacks of a mental illness diagnosis but none of the benefits. The diagnosis had a negative impact on access to services, on identity and hope, and was most associated with institutionalised stigma within mental health services.

Given that a diagnosis is supposed to enable help, care and treatment this is a curious finding, and one criticism of personality disorder as a diagnosis is that it does not capture the essence of the troubles that people experience. Because of this, some advocate the use of post-traumatic stress disorder as a diagnosis instead, given the link with trauma. Hong, Ilardi and Lishner (2011) state that 80% of those diagnosed with a personality disorder report adverse childhood experiences. Although it is reasonable to say that not all people who experience trauma growing up will go on to be diagnosed with a personality disorder and that, as this figure shows, not everyone who has been given this diagnosis has experienced traumatic early experiences, this is nonetheless a significant consideration.

Researchers at the University of Oxford, among others worldwide, report evidence showing that trauma leads to changes in the brain (Stark *et al.*, 2015), and Siegel (2012) contends that this means that the interaction between the social, personal and biological aspects have to be considered.

The NHS promotes the use of talking therapies as a treatment for people who have been given a diagnosis of personality disorder. Talking therapies are discussed in more detail in *Chapter 6*, but it is important to acknowledge here that health care professionals do not need to be trained in therapy to have a positive impact on people's experiences when accessing health care. Sweeney *et al.* (2018) discuss the importance of shifting thinking from 'What is wrong with you?' to considering 'What happened to you?' This shift, as well as an appreciation of the part neurobiology plays in relation to the experience of trauma, can help health care professionals to take a more empathic approach in understanding the presentation of people with a diagnosis of personality disorder when attending services, the importance of which is so clearly detailed by Perkins *et al.* (2018), as discussed above.

CHAPTER SUMMARY

Key points to take away from *Chapter 4*:

- ☑ We do not either have mental health difficulties or not have them; for all of us, mental health lies on a continuum and we can experience mental health difficulties at different times throughout our lives. Accepting this is one way to help develop empathy, which is one of the most important aspects of care when someone's mental health is affected.

- ☑ Therapeutic interventions and treatments for mental health difficulties are likely to be multifaceted. This is unlike a difficulty with a primary physical cause, which may have one specific recommended treatment, because mental health difficulties require a holistic approach that takes account of all dimensions of the person and must also account for those who are important to the person.

- ☑ Contrary to popular belief, it is not always required to have in-depth mental health training to be helpful. Often an empathic approach that shows understanding and a desire to intervene in a thoughtful, person-centred way makes a huge contribution and can be the difference between someone wanting to use health services and avoiding them even when they are desperately needed.

Questions

Question 4.1   Consider the mental health difficulties presented in this chapter and reflect on your own experiences, with the aim of developing your understanding and empathy. *(Learning outcome 4.1)*

Question 4.2   Taking a holistic perspective, consider the wide-ranging impact that mental health difficulties can have for a person across the life course. *(Learning outcome 4.2)*

Question 4.3   How will you know when a referral to a health care professional educated in therapeutic mental health interventions is required, and what skills and knowledge will you require to ensure that people are prepared for this and ease of access is facilitated? *(Learning outcome 4.3)*

FURTHER READING

Mental Health Foundation (2020) *How to... Overcome Fear and Anxiety.* Available at: www.mentalhealth.org.uk/sites/default/files/How%20to... fear%20and%20anxiety.pdf (accessed 23 June 2021).

Mental Health Foundation (2020) *How to... Look after Your Mental Health.* Available at: www.mentalhealth.org.uk/sites/default/files/How%20to... mental%20health.pdf (accessed 23 June 2021).

NHS (2020) *Mental Health Conditions.* Available at: www.nhs.uk/mental-health/conditions (accessed 23 June 2021).

NHS (2020) *Feelings, Symptoms and Behaviours.* Available at: www.nhs.uk/mental-health/feelings-symptoms-behaviours (accessed 23 June 2021).

Norman, I. and Ryrie, I. (eds) (2018) *The Art and Science of Mental Health Nursing: principles and practice*, 4th edition. Open University Press.

Time to Change (2020) *Personal Stories.* Available at: www.time-to-change.org.uk/personal-stories (accessed 23 June 2021).

Chapter 5
Mental health in early life

Celeste Foster and Eunice Ayodeji

LEARNING OUTCOMES

By the end of this chapter you should be able to:

5.1 Understand the relationship between mental health problems and child development

5.2 Describe the legal framework that guides working with children and young people who have mental health needs

5.3 Begin to recognise common mental health problems and signs of distress in children and young people

5.4 Reflect on the approaches, skills and knowledge that you can use to support children and young people in distress

5.5 Describe children's mental health services and referral pathways.

5.1 Introduction

Why are mental health, wellbeing and disorder in children and young people important?

People often wonder how it is that children and adolescents develop mental health problems. 'What have children got to be sad, upset or worried about? They're just kids, right? They don't have adult responsibilities or problems': these are commonly expressed views. There is also an understandable debate in our society about whether we are over-labelling ordinary emotional issues in childhood as psychiatric problems, and whether society is encouraging children to feel as though there is something wrong with them, when in fact they are just experiencing ordinary life problems.

The answer to these questions and concerns lies somewhere in the middle. It is important to stress that most children are living in good-enough circumstances and that, from a psychological perspective, they are thriving and growing as they should. Most children will also have emotional difficulties of some kind at some point in their childhood; but they will develop and grow through these difficulties, as they draw on the support of good-enough parents/carers, wider social support and their own internal resources, to overcome or resolve any problems life throws their way.

However, for a much smaller but equally important proportion of children and young people this is not the case. They are experiencing circumstances, life events or relationships that trigger significant amounts of mental distress which, without additional help and support, will get worse and lead to serious mental health problems.

It is estimated that in the UK one in five children and young people are experiencing emotional or behavioural problems at any one time (Deighton *et al.*, 2018), with one in eight children aged between 5 and 19 years having had at least one mental disorder (NHS Digital, 2018).

The evidence shows that children, and adolescents especially, who are experiencing mental distress are at risk of two problems. They can either be too quickly labelled as having a severe mental health problem and referred to specialist mental health services before they need it, causing them to feel stigmatised. Alternatively, their difficulties can be underestimated and dismissed as being 'ordinary teenager stuff', meaning they do not get the help they need at the time they need it. In both cases it can lead to problems getting much worse or lasting for much longer.

Since 1995, the prevalence of long-standing mental health conditions in children and young people (aged 4–24 years) has consistently increased (Pitchforth *et al.*, 2018). Globally, depression causes the biggest burden of ill health in children and young people (Patton *et al.*, 2016). Suicide is a leading cause of death for young people in the UK and the rate has not declined in 30 years (ONS, 2019). It is estimated that up to 75% of adult mental health conditions have their onset before the age of 24 (Kessler *et al.*, 2005).

So, we can see from the research evidence that responding in a timely way and providing early help for children and young people is important, not just for individual young people, but for the health and wellbeing of the whole population and future generations.

Perhaps understandably to some extent, professionals who come into contact with children and young people as part of their everyday work can be reluctant to respond to their mental health needs, beyond making referrals to specialist child and adolescent mental health services (CAMHS) – worrying that they do not have the skills or that they might make things worse. However, children's mental health is everyone's business. By understanding a little bit about child development and the factors that promote resilience, the law in relation to children, common signs of mental distress and how specialist services for children work, everyone can respond to children in a way that is helpful.

ACTIVITY 5.1

Being bullied is a negative life experience, not a mental health problem. However, the effects of either being bullied or doing the bullying, especially if persistent, have been shown to be directly linked to depression, anxiety, self-harm and suicidality in childhood. The effects last well into early adulthood, affecting occupational, financial, health and social outcomes (Copeland et al., 2013).

Consider the above statement in relation to your own area of practice. In what ways could you act to help a child you come into contact with who is being bullied or involved in bullying to try to reduce the chances of these long-term negative effects?

5.2 The link between child mental health and child development

Mental health and illness in children and teenagers are intimately linked to child development. The primary job of a child is to grow and develop towards becoming an adult; hopefully, along the way they will acquire the skills, resources and resilience that are needed to manage the stresses and strains of adult life successfully.

In good-enough circumstances, children are supported and enabled through each stage of development by positive attachment relationships in which they feel a sense of safety and belonging, and in which their physical, emotional and psychological needs are understood and met (Bowlby, 1988). In time, these relationships help the child to develop their own coping skills, sense of esteem and ability to understand and regulate their emotions, leading to a gradual move towards independence. Although attachment relationships are often thought of mostly as being with parents/primary carers, as the child gets older the number of significant relationships widens to include adults and peers in their broader family and community and in the systems and organisations in which they live and learn (Waddell, 2018).

It is widely agreed (NHS Health Advisory Service, 1995, p. 15) that good mental health in children and young people is indicated by:

- a capacity to enter into and sustain mutually satisfying personal relationships
- continuing progression of psychological development
- an ability to play and to learn, so that attainments are appropriate for age and intellectual level
- a developing moral sense of right and wrong
- the degree of psychological distress and maladaptive behaviour being within normal limits for the child's age and context.

What is important in this definition is the idea that children should not be expected to be happy all the time (even though as adults we might want that for them). Instead, they should be able to feel and express a full range of emotions that correspond to the circumstances that they are in. Ordinary learning and play activities are also essential to fostering good mental health in children, as they help young people maintain connections with their peers and help to foster positive identity formation, self-esteem and interpersonal skill development (Suris, Michaud and Viner, 2004).

Just as ordinary life events and relationships promote wellbeing and resilience in children, the experience of adverse life events can put children and young people's mental wellbeing at risk (Hughes *et al.*, 2017). Mental distress in children and young people is most commonly a response to what is happening within the systems in which they live (Scott, Arney and Vimpani, 2010). It is important to understand that this also includes the physiological systems of their own bodies. With the right support many children grow and thrive in the context of having a learning disability or long-term physical condition. However, significant physical illness, injury or disability, without appropriate support and adaptations from adults around them, can significantly disrupt ordinary social and emotional development for children. Similarly, although the developmental stage of adolescence is characterised by growth, creativity and opportunity for most young people, managing the uncertainty of the physical changes of puberty along with the increased social and educational demands and responsibilities makes adolescence a time of higher risk of onset of mental health problems (WHO, 2020).

Positive attachment relationships serve as a protection against the impact of some adverse childhood experiences, helping children to feel safe, bounce back and understand what has happened to them. However, if there is insufficient support and help for carers, some forms of childhood adversity can also have a negative impact on carers' abilities to provide care and safety for their children, further adding to the risks that children face. Helping children with mental health needs should therefore always be a whole-family approach. This involves promoting the wellbeing of all family members; maximising safety for the child; and at the same time supporting and empowering parents/carers to maximise their parenting capacity and the quality of their relationships with their children (Social Care Institute for Excellence, 2009).

ACTIVITY 5.2

Consider the impact of domestic violence or parental substance misuse on children and their primary carers. What kind of support could be provided for the child and for the carer?

Understanding the mental health needs of children and young people from the perspective of their developmental tasks and the system that they live in has several implications.

Firstly, the criteria for diagnosing mental illness were developed based on adults, and so children do not easily fit into them. This means that children and young people can look as though they have multiple mental health conditions (comorbidity). Alternatively, although they may have a high level of need, their difficulties may be hard to label using the diagnostic system. As children and young people are also always growing, learning and changing, the nature of their difficulties can seem to change often.

Secondly, children's mental health problems are most likely to be a response to difficulties in their life or to difficulties for which they have not yet had time to develop coping skills. There is therefore a much lower use of medicine-based treatments than in adult mental health services and a much stronger focus on social, psychological and skill-building interventions.

Lastly, in this model, expressing emotional upset and worry though challenging or changed behaviour is considered to be the normal way for children to communicate and cope with their difficulties. This is because they do not have fully developed language for emotional expression, or the cognitive skills needed to manage the stress they are experiencing. Problematic behaviour should be seen as holding information about how the child is feeling, viewed in the context of what is happening in their life and understood as functional (i.e. serving a purpose). When understood in this way, it becomes much easier to engage with children and young people and to help them think about alternative, more positive ways of managing their distress.

5.3 Underlying principles of child mental health service provision in the UK

In 2017, the UK government produced a green paper called *Transforming Children and Young People's Mental Health Provision* (Department of Health and Department of Education, 2017). As part of the changes being implemented to improve mental health service access for children and young people, a new model has been introduced called the THRIVE model (Wolpert *et al.*, 2014). In the past, children's mental health service pathways have been organisation-focused, whereas THRIVE is a child-focused model.

The THRIVE model works by (1) assuming that most children are thriving but will need some level of ongoing adult support to maintain this, (2) identifying children who are in need of additional help and the level of help they need at that time, then (3) matching them to the right sorts of intervention that different services provide. This recognises that several different services may be contributing to meeting a child's needs, not just health services. It also allows for the idea that children's level of need can change and that this is not always based on the presence of a mental health condition – many children have a diagnosis of a mental or a physical health condition, but with the right treatment and support can be thriving.

Embedded in the government's policies for children's mental health provision is the principle that all professionals, including non-mental health professionals, who come into contact with children, young people and their families have a role to play in early identification of children who need help. They should be able to fulfil this role by identifying children who are vulnerable, providing a helpful first response, access to information and guidance, and signposting to appropriate services (Department of Health and Department of Education, 2017).

To help make this principle a reality and to provide services for children as early as possible in the places in which they usually live and learn, services are being reorganised to make sure that access to mental health and wellbeing support is linked to schools and colleges. This includes the creation of a new role called education mental health practitioners (EMHPs). Education mental health practitioners work across education and health care to provide mental health support for children and young people in schools and colleges.

ACTIVITY 5.3

All professionals are expected to be able to contribute to children and young people's mental health in four areas: (1) identifying children who are vulnerable; (2) providing a helpful first response; (3) providing access to information and guidance; (4) signposting to appropriate services.

Which of these areas do you feel confident in and which do you feel you need to work on developing? Write yourself an action plan to help you build the skills and knowledge needed.

5.4 Understanding the legal framework for working with children and young people with mental health needs

In the UK, the legal framework for the care of children and young people is based on some key concepts:

- The welfare of the child is paramount in all decision-making processes.
- Children and young people are vulnerable due to their developmental immaturity, and so adults owe them a duty of care.
- Children and young people have the ability and right to express their wishes and feelings and participate in decisions about their life.
- Children and young people have the right to (limited) privacy and confidentiality, as long as this does not leave them in danger.
- All agencies, and the people who work for those agencies, have a responsibility to address the needs of children and their families at an early stage, and to identify and help those who are most vulnerable.

The amount of confidentiality and decision-making power a child or young person has depends on an interaction between their age, their level of cognitive maturity, and the type and magnitude of the decision that needs to be made. The main laws that govern this are the Children Act 1989 and 2004, the Mental Capacity Act 2005, the United Nations Convention on the Rights of the Child (UNCRC) (1989), the Human Rights Act 1998 and UK case law relating to the concept of 'Gillick competence'.

The Children Acts of 1989 and 2004 set out the rights of all children under UK law, the responsibilities of parents and carers to protect and maintain the welfare of their children up until their 18th birthday, and the responsibilities of the state when this goes wrong. Under the Mental Capacity Act 2005 and the Family Law Reform Act 1969, once a child reaches their 16th birthday, they are assumed to have the capacity to make informed decisions about their own welfare and treatment without being overridden, in the same way as adults. However, the situation is complex, as parents and carers still have a legal responsibility under the Children Act 1989 to protect and look after their children until they are 18 years old. Therefore, decision-making in relation to consent, confidentiality and information sharing for 16- and 17-year-olds can be complicated, especially when there are risks involved. It is important to seek guidance from someone in your organisation with expertise in this area on a case-by-case basis.

Decision-making for children who are under 16 is governed by the interaction between two concepts: 'the zone of parental control' (ZPC), sometimes referred to as the 'scope of parental responsibility' (SPR); and the relative competence of the child. Broadly speaking, as a child ages and matures, the zone of parental control diminishes and the rights and autonomy of the child increase, as their level of competence increases.

The ZPC/SPR covers decisions that a person with parental responsibility would ordinarily be expected to make, having regard for what is considered normal in our society, whether the parent/carer is acting in the child's best interests, and the developing cognitive maturity of the child. A Gillick-competent child is defined by law as one who has sufficient understanding and intelligence to enable them to fully understand and weigh up what is involved in the decision they are making and the likely consequences of any decision taken. This means that the competence of a child under 16 years must be assessed on a decision-by-decision basis and on each occasion that the decision needs to be made, as a child's competence can fluctuate from day to day.

If a child is Gillick-competent and gives consent, it is not necessary to gain consent from the person with parental responsibility. However, it is good practice to involve the parents/carers in the process if the child consents. Similarly, if a child is not competent and the parent/carer must make a decision, then the Children Act 1989 and the UNCRC say that we must ensure the child is involved in the decision-making process in the fullest way possible and that their wishes and preferences are given due weight in matters that affect them.

It is important to understand that having a mental health problem or disorder does not automatically mean that a child can be deemed to be without competence or capacity to make decisions. The presence of a mental disorder would only indicate that a formal assessment of the child's capacity/competence in relation to the decision in hand should be undertaken, in accordance with the appropriate guidelines (Department of Health, 2001; Mental Capacity Act 2005).

The Children Act 1989 also ensures that a child's wishes for confidentiality can be overruled in any case where the child is at risk of significant harm and that not sharing information would add to the risk of harm occurring. This is commonly referred to as safeguarding and detailed guidance about safeguarding responsibilities can be found in *Working Together to Safeguard Children* (Department for Education, 2018).

As an additional measure to safeguard children and young people in cases where parents/carers cannot be relied on to act in their child's best interests, every child and young person up to the age of 18 is subject to the inherent jurisdiction of the High Court, which can overrule parental authority in specific cases.

ACTIVITY 5.4

To assess whether a child has Gillick competence to make a decision you must be able to check that they can understand the decision to be made, weigh up the information needed to make the decision and understand the consequences of the decision.

Reflect on the communication skills you would need to use and the steps you would need to take to check for Gillick competence in practice.

5.5 Common mental health conditions in children and young people

5.5.1 Depression

Depression is one of the most common mental health problems in children and young people and it is rarely uncomplicated. It can cause considerable distress and can have a profound impact on the young person and their family/carers. Depression is uncommon in very young children (before puberty), with prevalence rates of 1–2%, rising to 20% in adolescence (Avenevoli *et al.*, 2015; Costello, Erkanli and Angold, 2006). Rates of depression vary between boys and girls, with a higher incidence in girls, a gender difference that persists into adulthood (Angold and Costello, 2001). For a diagnosis of depression young people must fulfil at least five out of nine symptoms:

- loss of interest or pleasure
- low mood or irritability
- decrease or increase in sleep
- decreased or increased appetite or weight
- agitation
- fatigue
- poor concentration
- feelings of worthlessness
- suicidal thoughts or plans.

One of the two core symptoms – marked diminished interest/pleasure in almost all activities, or low mood/irritability – must be present at all times. Most young people (especially adolescents) experience periods of sadness and despondency, making it difficult to identify depression in this population. The clinical presentation and symptoms of depression in children and young people are similar to those seen in the adult population; however, children are not 'mini adults' and symptoms and presentation are dependent on the young person's developmental stage, and clear developmental differences exist between childhood and adolescent depression. For example, younger children may present with tummy aches, whereas older children may present as bored, irritable and oversleeping.

Table 5.1 outlines some common misconceptions about depression in young people.

Table 5.1 *Myths about depression in children and adolescents*

Myth	Fact
Depression/moodiness is normal in teenagers	Persistent low mood is not normal. They can't just 'snap out of it'. It's not 'just the hormones'.
Children and adolescents are mini adults	Childhood and adolescent depression is different from adult depression.
Discussing depression/suicidality with children and adolescents may make things worse	There is no evidence that discussing depression/suicidality will increase suicidal behaviour. It is often a relief for the child.
It is important that parents should continue to strictly enforce behavioural consequences with depressed children and adolescents	Overly strict parenting may not be helpful and can further lower self-esteem. Depressed children and adolescents will struggle with school/activities; parents need to choose their battles and to support and encourage with appropriate boundaries.
Antidepressants are unsuitable for teenagers	Antidepressants can be useful in moderate to severe depression in adolescents, but rarely as first line treatment (especially in children). They should always be prescribed and monitored by a child psychiatrist.

5.5.2 Anxiety

Worries are a normal part of child and adolescent development, and most young people will experience episodes of worry or will feel fearful from time to time. The ways in which children and young people express their anxiety change in relation to their stage of development. For example, in young children anxiety is usually caused by fears of strangers and/or separation from their primary caregivers, fears of the dark and of imaginary creatures. In adolescence anxiety is commonly provoked by fear of social situations and performance anxiety. These worries and fears, although unpleasant, can also be helpful as they can prepare our body to respond to danger or attack in an appropriate way. However, if these fears and worries are intense, they can have a significant impact on the young person's day-to-day functioning, and the young person may experience worrying thoughts and fears constantly. Many children and young people experience anxiety, and it is one of the most common mental health difficulties in childhood and adolescence. Anxiety can co-occur with depression, and this makes it difficult to state the numbers for anxiety alone. However, figures from the Royal College of Psychiatrists (RCPsych) indicate that in 2015 approximately 300,000 children and young people in Britain had an anxiety disorder (www.rcpsych.ac.uk/mental-health/parents-and-young-people/young-people/worries-and-anxieties).

Anxiety conditions in children and young people

Anxiety problems specific to childhood:
- separation anxiety
- phobic anxiety specific to childhood
- social anxiety specific to childhood.

Phobic anxiety:
- agoraphobia
- social phobia.

Other anxiety conditions:
- panic disorder
- generalised anxiety disorder
- mixed anxiety and depressive disorder.

ACTIVITY 5.5

Describe/define the anxiety conditions in children and young people in *Section 5.5.2*. You can find information by accessing any of the websites in the resources section at the end of this chapter.

5.5.3 Neurodevelopmental conditions

Neurodevelopmental conditions are differences in the development and functioning of the brain that can affect a child's behaviour, memory or ability to learn. These differences tend to be lifelong. However, children and adults are always learning and growing, and so changes and improvements do occur. Attention deficit hyperactivity disorder (ADHD) and autism spectrum disorder (ASD) are both classed as neurodevelopmental conditions.

Attention deficit hyperactivity disorder (ADHD)

Many children are inattentive, impulsive and hyperactive. However, ADHD is characterised by developmentally inappropriate and exaggerated inattention, hyperactivity and impulsiveness. These characteristics typically start in early to mid childhood (WHO, 2019a), and consequently the symptoms typically cause problems in the school, home and community environments and they can also be associated with behavioural problems. ADHD is more common in boys than girls, with a prevalence ratio of around 4:1. NICE advises that first line treatment for this condition following diagnosis should be psychoeducation about the conditions and strategies to manage the symptoms. In most cases, children are prescribed the stimulant medication methylphenidate (NCCMH, 2018b), which can reduce symptoms of hyperactivity and inattention, improving focus and performance at school. However, every child's response to stimulant medication is individual, so each child has to be closely monitored to check for side effects and whether the benefits outweigh the risks of this medicine.

Autism spectrum disorder (ASD)

As the name suggests, autism spectrum disorder is a spectrum and there are considerable variations with regard to presentation, from mild to severe. The prevalence rate is between 1.2 and 2% (Elsabbagh *et al.*, 2012). This condition also includes Asperger syndrome, a name given to describe children who have the features of autism but without any associated learning disability or problems acquiring language. Children who experience autism spectrum conditions usually have difficulties in three main areas:
1. impairment in social interaction
2. restricted, repetitive interests and behaviour
3. impairment in communication.

Children who experience this condition can be vulnerable to other mental health problems, such as ADHD and anxiety, and often experience behavioural difficulties.

5.5.4 Self-harm

Self-harm in adolescence is a serious and increasing problem, with many young people either directly engaging in episodes of self-harm or knowing another young person who has self-harmed. There is an ongoing debate in relation to what constitutes self-harm. Self-harm can include behaviours such as over-eating and engaging in high-risk activities such as harmful alcohol and drug misuse. NICE (2011c) suggests that self-harm can involve self-poisoning, or self-injury (including cutting, taking an overdose, hanging, self-strangulation, jumping from a height, and running into traffic), irrespective of motivation or intent. Although not a diagnosis, self-harm often co-occurs with other mental health conditions; it most frequently occurs with depression, and approximately two-thirds of young people who self-harm also have depression (Cloutier *et al.*, 2010).

A seven-country European collaborative study highlighted that self-harm is a common problem in this international community (Madge *et al.*, 2008). Worryingly, the evidence suggests that 10% of young people who self-harm will repeat this behaviour within six months and 42% will repeat it within 21 months (Brent *et al.*, 1993).

The Health Behaviour in School-Aged Children report (Brooks *et al.*, 2015) surveyed 6,000 UK school children aged 11, 13 and 15. Questions in relation to self-harming behaviour were asked of the 15-year-olds only, and 20% reported that they had previously self-harmed. Between 2012/2013 and 2018/2019, hospital admissions following self-harm rose by 36% for females aged 10–24, whereas the rate for males remained roughly constant (Nuffield Trust, 2020).

The reasons that young people self-harm are varied and are different for each individual. Typically, it can be understood as an expression of distress, an attempt to cope with overwhelming feelings or experiences, or a response to frightening or stressful life events. Helping young people who self-harm involves understanding the underlying causes for the individual, addressing these wherever possible and helping the young person find safer ways of coping with their feelings.

5.5.5 Psychotic experiences in young people

Chapter 4 gives a detailed outline of psychotic illnesses such as schizophrenia. The onset of psychosis in children and young people is relatively uncommon. Young people who do develop these conditions are cared for by specialist multidisciplinary teams called early intervention teams (EITs). However, hearing voices as a single symptom without the presence of a psychotic illness is something that can happen to quite a lot of children and young people. Research studies have estimated that between 10 and 17% of children and young people hear a voice that they do not think is their own at some point in their childhood or adolescence, and only about 5% find the experiencing troubling (Kompus *et al.*, 2015). Troubling experiences of hearing voices for children and young people are much more often a symptom of acute anxiety, stress or drug use, or are associated with memories of frightening events, rather than onset of severe mental illness such as schizophrenia.

5.5.6 Vulnerable groups

Mental health problems have the potential to develop in all children. However, there are specific groups of children who are more vulnerable to developing mental health problems. There are several known psychosocial risk factors that can increase the likelihood of mental health difficulties. In addition, belonging to certain populations can make a young person more vulnerable to developing mental health difficulties (Hughes *et al.*, 2017). However, it is important to understand that the risk associated with belonging to an identified vulnerable group is largely because of the increased risk of being excluded, marginalised and discriminated against, and of having to access health services that do not understand the individual's needs, rather than from belonging to the group itself (Department of Health and Department of Education, 2017). *Table 5.2* highlights risk factors associated with child mental health difficulties, and groups that have been identified as particularly vulnerable. To balance out the risk factors, there are also resilience factors (Collishaw *et al.*, 2016), which can cushion and protect the young person from developing mental health difficulties or decrease the severity of a mental health problem. These resilience factors include, among others:

- positive expressed emotion (EE) in the main parent
- co-parent support
- good quality social relationships
- self-efficacy
- frequent exercise.

Many children and young people will belong to more than one of the vulnerable groups. Furthermore, they may experience multiple risk factors. However, it is unclear whether there is a cumulative effect.

Table 5.2 *Risk factors for developing mental health problems and vulnerable groups*

Risk factors	Vulnerable populations
• Parental mental illness • Personal history of mental illness • More than three stressful life events • Family discord • Adversity and trauma • Drug and alcohol misuse • Medical problems (serious and chronic illnesses) • Learning disabilities • Physical disabilities • Bullying • Deprivation • Discrimination • Authoritarian parenting • Academic demands • Poor sleep • Homelessness • Living in institutional settings	• LGBTQ+ youth • Refugee status • Black, Asian and other ethnic minority communities • Children in care and looked-after children • Children in traveller communities • Young people involved in gangs

5.6 Specialist child and adolescent mental health services (CAMHS)

CAMHS professionals often deal with a broad range of complex mental health problems, including all the difficulties/conditions outlined above. They are trained and experienced in identifying (assessing), understanding, managing and treating (using evidence-based interventions) young people who present to services with mental health difficulties. One key difference between CAMHS and adult mental health services is the way in which treatments are delivered. Professionals working in CAMHS must be able to adapt evidence-based interventions in a way that is suitable for the child's age, stage of development and abilities. This often involves using strategies that mirror how children usually learn – for example, using play, activities, experiential or structured learning strategies – and for younger children especially, it often involves parents and carers. *Table 5.3* outlines the roles and responsibilities of the core professionals who work in CAMHS, and some of the interventions they can provide. These may be offered on their own (unidisciplinary) for children with moderate difficulties, or in conjunction with other members of the team (multidisciplinary) in more complex or severe cases.

Table 5.3 *Roles and responsibilities in CAMHS*

Mental health nurses	Skilled in the assessment and treatment of children with complex, acute and enduring mental health problems. Provide extensive support for both the young person and their parents/carers. Provide psychoeducation around the presenting symptoms and the management of the mental health condition.
Mental health practitioners	Come from a wide variety of professional backgrounds and support members of the CAMHS team in the assessment, management and treatment of a wide variety of mental health, emotional and behavioural difficulties.
Social workers	Contribute to the assessment of children and young people experiencing mental health problems and help to strengthen links between CAMHS and other children and young people's services. They are particularly skilled in supporting other members of the CAMHS team to develop an understanding of vulnerable groups, e.g. looked-after children, and in supporting families and carers.
Clinical psychologists	Use a variety of assessment tools to gain an understanding of the social, behavioural and emotional difficulties the child is experiencing and the resulting impact on the family. They are often asked to undertake a comprehensive psychological assessment and produce a report with recommendation for treatment. They provide evidence-based psychological interventions in accordance with NICE clinical guidelines.
Systemic family therapists	There are many different models of family therapy, and CAMHS family therapists usually work in a systemic way to assess the difficulties both within the family as a whole and between individual family members.
Child psychiatrists	Medically trained doctors who specialise in the diagnosis, medical treatment and management of children and young people with complex mental health problems. They often provide highly specialised advice/consultations and training to other agencies, in particular children's services, and they prescribe medicine when indicated.
Child psychotherapists	Utilise a variety of approaches to help the child explore and make sense of their inner world (thoughts, feelings, beliefs) in the context of the child's difficulties. They help children acquire new skills for coping with their difficulties.

ACTIVITY 5.6

Find out where your local CAMHS is and how you would make a referral to it, if you were worried about a child or young person.

5.6.1 When to refer to CAMHS?

This is not an easy question to answer, as it will need to be judged on a case-by-case basis. Local CAMHS can often help by providing advice about children you are worried about. They will probably want to know what has been tried so far to help the child, to make sure that the individual is not being referred to a specialist mental health service too quickly, when help from people they know might work better.

NICE (2011b) has produced some helpful questions to help you identify whether a referral to CAMHS might be needed:

- Are the risks associated with the mental health concerns increasing or unresponsive to my attempts to help?
- Are levels of distress rising, high or sustained?
- Has the young person requested further help from specialist services?
- Are levels of distress in parents or carers rising, high or sustained despite attempts to help?

Sustained changes in a child's developmental progression, learning and everyday functioning can also be a good indicator that more specialist help is needed.

5.7 Recognising signs of distress and responding helpfully

When you have recognised changes or behaviours in a child or young person that make you concerned, the most vital thing is to have a conversation with them. Let them know you are concerned in a non-critical way and that you are available to help. Don't be afraid to ask gentle questions about the child's thoughts and feelings; this will help you work out what to do next and when you need to seek advice and guidance. Children do not always know the answers to these questions though, so communicate in a way that does not show frustration.

Children and young people who have experienced adverse childhood events are likely to struggle with entering, establishing and maintaining therapeutic or helping relationships with adults. It is important to recognise that, because of their past experiences, the child or young person may not trust adults, and any attempts to help are likely to be sabotaged. It is important to be gently persistent in attempts to engage the young person – not to give up but not to be too intrusive.

Any strategies that help the child make sense of their experiences and support and strengthen carer–child relationships will be helpful. Practical strategies that reduce stresses on parents are also beneficial. Equipping yourself with knowledge of local organisations and support services for children and their families will help you to help them.

Remember always to seek advice and support from within your organisation about any child or young person who is causing you concern.

5.7.1 Top tips for helping children and young people who are experiencing mental distress

Talking to children and young people

- Children and young people experiencing mental health problems need a safe, calm and secure environment.
- Promote a structured day with a balance between activities and relaxation, between work and play.
- Be reliable and consistent; try not to offer more than you can deliver.
- Use clear verbal communication that conveys interest in the child.
- Be clear about the limits of confidentiality.
- Acknowledge and validate their distress, and always take their concerns seriously.
- Demonstrate an attitude of acceptance and curiosity.
- Ask direct questions when seeking specific information.
- Use age-appropriate language.
- Remember that behaviour is information; demonstrate acceptance and interest in understanding the child's behaviour, to promote a trusting therapeutic relationship.
- Collaborate with the young person to reach a shared understanding of their mental health difficulties.
- Remain calm at all times.

Helping children with their difficulties

- Normalise the mental health difficulties the young person is experiencing by putting them in context and indicating to the young person that they are not alone in experiencing them.
- Provide psychoeducation in relation to their mental health problem and strategies to help them manage their distress.
- Signpost to good quality sources of self-help (see resources in the 'Further reading' at the end of this chapter).
- Support children and young people to go through structured problem-solving approaches to address the things that are causing them stress/distress.
- Collaborate with the young person about the supports that will be put in place.
- Help the child engage in meaningful activities that bring pleasure, a sense of achievement and self-efficacy, including considering reasonable adjustments in school.

5.7.2 The nurse's role in supporting children and young people with mental health problems/difficulties

Nurses comprise the biggest professional group in the NHS and CAMHS, and are often the first point of contact when a parent, carer, teacher or GP is worried about a child's mental health. Owing to the increase in mental health problems within the child and adolescent population, nurses in many fields are likely to come across young people who are experiencing mental health difficulties. Therefore, it is essential that they are equipped with the relevant information to know how to respond helpfully to the young person and their family.

CHAPTER SUMMARY

Key points to take away from *Chapter 5*:

☑ Mental health and wellbeing across the life course are influenced by early life experiences and relationships. The balance of positive and adverse experiences in a child's life, and the ways in which they are helped to make sense and cope with any difficulties, contribute to their unique mix of resilience and vulnerability.

☑ Early/timely support for children experiencing mental distress can help resolve difficulties before they become a serious mental health problem. Wherever possible, help is best delivered by people that the child or young person knows well, rather than specialist services.

☑ Expressing emotional distress through behaviour is developmentally normal for children and young people. Taking time to understand the context and function of behaviour, and helping children put their behaviour, feelings and worries into words, form a cornerstone of helping children to recover from mental health difficulties.

☑ Treatment for mental disorder in children and young people should always consider the needs of the whole family and include strategies to support parents/carers to be the most effective parents/carers they can be.

Questions

Question 5.1	Describe the relationship between mental health and child development. (*Learning outcome 5.1*)
Question 5.2	What are the characteristics that tell you a child has competence to make a particular decision? (*Learning outcome 5.2*)
Question 5.3	List the most common types of mental health problem for children and the signs and symptoms that would indicate that a child is experiencing problems. (*Learning outcome 5.3*)
Question 5.4	Develop a list of the ways in which you can contribute to helping children who are experiencing mental distress and their carers/family, based on what you have learnt. (*Learning outcome 5.4*)
Question 5.5	Identify the different professionals who are commonly involved in the care of a young person who is experiencing a mental health problem. (*Learning outcome 5.5*)

FURTHER READING

Griffith, R. (2016) What is Gillick competence? *Human Vaccines & Immunotherapuetics*, **12(1)**: 244–247.

NHS Inform (2020) *Anxiety Disorders in Children*. Available at: www.nhsinform.scot/illnesses-and-conditions/mental-health/anxiety-disorders-in-children (accessed 23 June 2021).

ONLINE RESOURCES

MindEd is a free online learning resource on children and young people's mental health, for all adults. It is funded by the Department of Health and the Department of Education (www.minded.org.uk).

The Royal College of Psychiatrists provides plain English leaflets and information for children and adults about common childhood mental health problems (www.rcpsych.ac.uk/mental-health/parents-and-young-people).

YoungMinds is a national charity that campaigns and provides resources to support and enable the emotional wellbeing of young people and their parents/carers. It has a range of resources and information for young people and adults on its website, and a telephone helpline for parents (youngminds.org.uk).

Chapter 6
Mental health in adulthood

Lorna McGlynn, Neil Murphy and Shelly Allen

LEARNING OUTCOMES

By the end of this chapter you should be able to:

6.1 Define therapeutic interventions used to support mental health in adulthood

6.2 Discuss the roles and responsibilities of professionals who deliver those interventions

6.3 Explore the range and scope of mental health service provision for adults

6.4 Examine the links between mental and physical health

6.5 Describe mental health provision within contemporary health care.

6.1 Introduction

This chapter reviews evidence-based interventions that are used to support mental health in adulthood. It then moves on to detail the roles and responsibilities of professionals who are involved in the delivery of those interventions, in conjunction with the context in which such care takes place.

6.2 Interventions

6.2.1 Care Programme Approach

The Care Programme Approach (CPA) was introduced in 1991 to improve the coordination of care for people with severe mental illness and it is a key mental health policy in England (Simpson, Miller and Bowers, 2003). The CPA is a framework used to direct the assessment, care, support, planning and review of people referred to secondary care mental health services.

The CPA is based on good practice within mental health services and it involves a multidisciplinary team, who provide care and support to people with severe mental illness (SMI). The CPA is aimed at adults of working age requiring mental health services and can include many types of service, such as community mental health services and inpatient mental health services. The CPA requires every patient to have a comprehensive care plan highlighting their needs and the requirements of services involved in delivering that care, such as clinical support and physical health needs. The person's care plan must be reviewed on a regular basis by all the professionals involved in their care (Goodwin and Lawton-Smith, 2010). A person under the CPA will be allocated a care coordinator, who is usually a nurse or social worker. This individual is responsible for the coordination and monitoring of the person's care; they will meet with the person on a regular basis to ensure that the person is remaining well and to review their care needs.

6.2.2 Medication

There are many different medications available for people with diagnosed mental health problems. This section will look at the groups commonly prescribed.

Antidepressants

This is the group of drugs that is the most frequently prescribed in the UK. There are several groups of compounds, but for ease of explanation we will explore one specifically: selective serotonin reuptake inhibitors (SSRIs) – for example, citalopram and fluoxetine. Owing to the chemical nature of these drugs, there is a delay in the active component reaching a therapeutic level (what is regarded as the optimum level in the body for some positive reaction). Most people taking SSRIs will not notice any benefit for around 14 days. During this period they may, however, experience associated side effects (e.g. tiredness, problems with sleep, headaches and difficulty concentrating).

These drugs work by limiting the messages sent by neurotransmitters to reabsorb serotonin (neurotransmitters are the chemicals the brain uses to communicate). Although regarded as good at 'lifting people's mood', and having evidence for treating anxiety problems as well, medication of this nature should not be prescribed before an accurate assessment of mood and a clinical identification of depression is made. This can mean that people may be expected to have experienced symptoms of depression for at least one month before diagnosis (WHO, 2019a).

Anxiolytics

Drugs in this group are frequently limited to short-term use owing to their habit-forming potential. The commonly prescribed drugs in this section are benzodiazepines (e.g. diazepam, lorazepam). The most common use of these drugs is to treat anxiety problems (e.g. generalised anxiety disorder, social phobia). Generally, anxiety-type presentations are initially treated with CBT, but in extreme situations, anxiolytics are prescribed for a short-term intervention. For this medication to be prescribed there is an anticipation that anxiety symptoms have been present over the preceding six months.

Anxiolytics work by increasing neurotransmitters in the brain. These chemicals include dopamine and serotonin. It is interesting to note that serotonin (especially) is linked to depression and that commonly both anxiety and depression often co-present in many people. Therefore, drugs that are effective have a similar neurotransmitter focus.

Antipsychotics

There is a range of drugs used to treat mental health problems with symptoms of psychotic experiences (e.g. schizophrenia). This group of drugs has various other names, such as neuroleptics and major tranquillisers. Essentially, most work through the blocking of dopamine, a neurotransmitter in the brain that helps pass messages on quickly. The key outcome of the use of antipsychotic drugs is to reduce the flow of messages facilitated by neurotransmitters. Antipsychotics affect the passage of serotonin (5-HT), commonly seen in the presentation of depressive type problems. Antipsychotic medication involves many receptors in the brain, but commonly the aim is to block some receptors and slow message transport.

The commonly prescribed antipsychotic drugs are from a family referred to as 'atypical' or 'second-generation' antipsychotics. These were developed in the 1990s, and they have fewer side effects than older drugs and are better tolerated. Instead of totally blocking neural receptors, these drugs transiently block pathways and quickly allow the dopamine transition to continue normally. Examples of these drugs include risperidone, quetiapine and aripiprazole.

The major problem with these drugs is their side effects, which are the most common reason for people ceasing to take them. A good list of drugs and their side effects can be found in the British National Formulary (BNF, updated twice per year) and on the Mind website (Mind, 2020), where impartial and clear advice is offered. Weight gain, type 2 diabetes, tiredness and QTc prolongation (when the heart takes longer than usual to recover after each beat) are possible.

These drugs are commonly administered orally, but there are some (e.g. aripiprazole) that can be given in a depot injection on a less frequent schedule (every 1–2 weeks). The major clinical concern related to these drugs is the potential of neuroleptic malignant syndrome (NMS). This is seen to a lesser extent with the second-generation antipsychotics, but it is still a concern and can occur after only one administration of the drug. NMS is characterised by further alteration to mental state, hyperthermia, autonomic instability and muscular rigidity, and the risk of death if NMS occurs is between 5 and 20%.

ACTIVITY 6.1

Consider occasions when you may not be able to use the BNF and consider what actions you could have taken before being placed in such a situation.

6.2.3 Motivational interviewing

Motivational interviewing is a therapeutic technique that was developed to support people who were experiencing problematic substance use. It aims to identify an individual's strengths and aspirations, helps capture the motivation for change and promotes autonomous decision-making (Rollnick *et al.*, 2008). During its development and as the underpinning evidence base grew, it began to be used more widely. This is illustrated in *Making Every Contact Count* (PHE, 2018a), which recommends motivational interviewing (although it does not use the term) in relation to the exploration of lifestyle risk factors such as diet, physical activity, tobacco use and alcohol. It is a good example of the integrated nature of mental and physical health, not just in relation to difficulties associated with lifestyle factors but also in productive attempts to address them.

Motivational interviewing rests on an understanding of change as a complex process that is not simply dependent on giving advice. Prochaska and DiClemente (1982) illustrated this with a cyclical model that considered the stages of change as *precontemplation, contemplation, preparation, action, maintenance* and *relapse*. This illustrates that change is not simply a linear process; it is dynamic, and the stages may have to be worked through numerous times before change can really be said to have been made.

ACTIVITY 6.2

Reflect on your experiences of being advised to do something you did not want to do, even though you knew it was for the best. Consider why it is that knowing the best or healthiest option in a given situation does not necessarily mean it will be chosen.

6.2.4 Talking therapies

This term refers to several approaches that include counselling and psychotherapy, and that have both differences and commonalities; for instance, all have the shared aim of helping us understand what troubles us. The Mental Health Foundation provides a list of talking therapies that can help in gaining an appreciation of the different approaches available (www.mentalhealth.org.uk/a-to-z/t/talking-therapies).

When considering different approaches to talking therapy, there is evidence to suggest that the nature of the relationship between therapist and client or patient is crucial (Ardito and Rabellino, 2011). It may therefore be reasonable to suggest that it is not that one therapy is better than another, but that it is the fit between the therapist, the approach and the individual that is crucial in effecting change.

That one therapy does not take precedence over another is also illustrated in the evidence base that underpins talking therapies. Computerised CBT, to be discussed later in this chapter, is one example of an intervention that comes under the umbrella term of talking therapies. Psychodynamic psychotherapy is another approach, which will now be considered more fully.

Psychodynamic psychotherapy

Psychodynamic psychotherapy is a therapeutic intervention that aims to help uncover the unconscious influences that are affecting the person's relationship with themselves and others. These influences are often hidden from us because they are painful and/or anxiety-provoking. In such circumstances a range of defence mechanisms serve to help keep them hidden from our conscious awareness.

A frequently used analogy to promote understanding of this is by reference to an iceberg. What can be seen on the surface is significant but is by no means the whole story, and what is occurring beneath, which cannot readily be seen without making an effort, is just as important. This means that for deep-seated change to occur, aspects of our mental life that are hidden need to be experienced and understood, and this is where psychodynamic psychotherapy aims to have an impact.

It can be an unsettling experience, but is one that can bring about a greater understanding of the self, relationships with others and why one continues to repeat some aspects of these even though they are unhelpful. Exploration of this is through what is referred to as the transference relationship with the psychotherapist. The British Psychoanalytic Council (BPC) explains this as unconscious patterns of the person's inner world, which are reflected in their relationship with the therapist (www.bpc.org.uk/information-support/what-is-therapy). The therapist then offers an interpretation of these for the person to consider. Promotion of understanding in this way can reduce distress and enhance insight.

Psychodynamic psychotherapy has been criticised for lacking an evidence base. However, this argument relies on a narrow definition of what constitutes evidence. If randomised controlled trials (RCTs) are seen as the only evidence worth considering, then this may be valid to an extent. However, there is a wealth of individual and clinician-reported evidence that supports this approach. Additionally, evaluation of psychodynamic psychotherapy in RCTs has become part of the growing evidence base for this therapy. There is evidence showing that the impact of psychodynamic psychotherapy is favourable at long-term follow-up and therefore goes beyond the treatment period, which enables lasting benefits. The BPC summarise the evidence on its website (www.bpc.org.uk/information-support/the-evidence-base).

6.2.5 Social prescribing

Social prescribing is defined by Health Education England (2016) as a range of non-clinical interventions that can help people to improve their wellbeing and resilience. Duffin (2016) also describes social prescribing as a non-clinical option for patients to improve their quality of life and wellbeing via a GP or other health care professional. The idea is that addressing areas such as physical activity, finances and relationships is just as important as addressing a person's physical health in order to improve their overall wellbeing (Husk *et al.*, 2019). Social prescribing provides a structured way to address the determinants of health and wellbeing for people accessing primary care and is integral to the NHS Long Term Plan (NHS, 2019).

There is growing evidence that social factors such as education, income and housing influence health behaviours and have a major impact on health (King's Fund, 2020). It is therefore equally important that people receive support for these factors in order to prevent ill health. Social prescribing interventions can include activities such as gardening, walking, social and art-based groups, volunteering, financial management and housing support. Referrals to social prescribing can be made by a person's GP, nurses and other health care professionals, via a link worker, who will spend time with the person, focusing on what matters to them, as identified through shared decision-making or personalised care and support planning (see www. england.nhs.uk/personalisedcare/social-prescribing). Link workers give advice and support to people who may benefit from social prescribing interventions, and they can link people with community groups and agencies for practical and emotional support. Such interventions are often identified as 'asset-based community services or groups' and they can be run by the voluntary or community sector (NHS England and NHS Improvement, 2019). A key target group for social prescribing is patients who have long-term mental/physical health conditions, are socially isolated and/ or require a greater level of social and emotional support to improve wellbeing and health (Drinkwater, Wildman and Moffatt, 2019).

Social prescribing goes hand in hand with 'signposting', which provides an infrastructure for connecting patients and the public to community services to address a range of health and social issues, and it is seen as a 'lighter touch'. As a nurse you can signpost people to services, using local knowledge and resource directories to identify the right professionals, services or activities. Active signposting works best for people who are confident and skilled enough to find their own way to services after a brief intervention (Health Education England, 2016).

ACTIVITY 6.3

Conduct an online search for your local area, to explore the different types of social prescribing activities and self-help interventions that you could signpost/refer your patients to.

6.2.6 Self-help

There have been several studies indicating that self-help interventions such as leaflets or letters have improved symptoms of depression in the short term; they also show that promoting effective self-help strategies early is just one way to help with depressive disorders (e.g. see Morgan, Jorm and Mackinnon, 2013). Self-help therapies are psychological therapies that people can use when experiencing mental health difficulties or poor mental wellbeing, using their own efforts without the aid of others. As a nurse you may encounter people with mild symptoms of depression and/or anxiety, so it would be useful to be aware of self-help interventions. Self-help might include help with anxiety, depression, obsessive–compulsive disorder and low self-esteem.

Textbooks that were originally designed for therapists were an early route to obtaining self-help, but a wide range of self-help books now enables people to explore therapeutic intervention without the help of a professional. Self-help interventions/therapies are also available to everyone in other forms, such as blogs, leaflets, audio books, online apps and tools, which are easily accessible online.

6.2.7 Computerised CBT

CBT is a set of therapeutic interventions traditionally conducted face to face with a therapist that aims to change the way that people think in order to develop alternative behaviours and emotional responses. There are many challenges for people accessing this help – for example, few therapists, long waiting lists, 'office hours' and client preference for the form of CBT (e.g. dialectical behavioural therapy, self-instructional training).

Not everyone feels that they can benefit from face-to-face therapy, as it does not fit into their lifestyle or their preferred way of seeking health care support, and the availability of the internet around the clock has become a draw for some looking for answers to their mental health problems. To cater for such people, a variety of companies and health care providers have developed electronic versions of CBT available on the internet. This was first explored in fairly simple yet interactive platforms such as Beating the Blues (www.beatingtheblues.co.uk), being further developed as information technology improved and there are now newer, more intuitive and less technical sites offering 'e-therapy', such as www.online-therapy.com.

The NHS has a web page where a number of mental health apps are listed and described: www.nhs.uk/apps-library/category/mental-health.

ACTIVITY 6.4

How would you feel about accessing help for a perceived problem from a computerised platform instead of from a professional?

6.3 Mental health services

6.3.1 Inpatient mental health environments

Inpatient mental health environments include hospitals and community inpatient settings such as rehabilitation units. All of these are facilities for people who may present a risk to themselves and/or others and who require extra support and monitoring in a safe environment where health professionals can assess them and provide interventions to help them. A range of health professionals work in inpatient units, including psychiatric nurses, occupational therapists, psychiatrists, psychologists, psychotherapists, and support, time and recovery (STR) workers.

People can be admitted on a voluntary basis or be detained under the Mental Health Act 1983. Patients will be provided with a range of treatments and interventions, such as medication, talking therapies and occupational therapy, depending on their identified needs. Mental health service provision should be needs-led, outcome-focused, responsive and delivered in a way that empowers people to build on their strengths, promotes recovery, supports families and carers, and ensures equality and fairness for all (NHS, 2018).

6.3.2 The independent sector

The Royal College of Nursing (RCN, 2013, p. 3) defines the independent sector as 'encompassing individuals, employers, and organisations [delivering] a broad spectrum of health and social care, who are wholly or partially independent of the public sector'. The health service utilises independent and voluntary organisations to provide services that the NHS is not able to, which may be due to a shortage or a lack of such services within the NHS (NHS Confederation, 2017). Although NHS mental health Trusts make up the largest single type of provider, there are other independent providers of mental health inpatient services and social care organisations offering community-based mental health care and/or learning disability services. These include commercial enterprises, and voluntary, charitable or not-for-profit organisations. Services and staff in the independent sector, such as hospitals and nursing homes, are regulated in the same way as NHS services via the Care Quality Commission (CQC), the Health and Safety Executive and professional bodies such as the General Medical Council (GMC) and the Nursing and Midwifery Council (NMC).

6.3.3 Primary care (Improving Access to Psychological Therapies)

Improving Access to Psychological Therapies (IAPT) services were first developed in 2008 in England to help address the needs of people experiencing anxiety and depression. In the *Five Year Forward View* (NHS England, 2014) IAPT was pivotal in the attempt to plan services that were proactive and avoided the deterioration of mental health due to untreated episodes.

IAPT services use evidence-based treatments and are generally provided by specialist and accredited staff with specialist knowledge of psychological interventions. The range of difficulties IAPT now supports includes, for example, anxiety, depression, PTSD and obsessive–compulsive behaviour.

The level of user involvement makes a lot of the therapy provided by IAPT services more realistic, utilising life events experienced or perceived to have been experienced and aiming to 'up-skill' the person seeking help. Commonly, the individual's symptoms are assessed at the start and end of treatment, so that they can see how helpful the intervention was. To further enhance the sense of involvement, routine monitoring is used in each session so the person involved in the treatment can self-monitor and understand the process of therapy and the changes that may well be happening with their problem.

Generally, there are two levels of IAPT service: low and high intensity. The level depends on the presentation and complexity of the client's difficulties. More time is generally given to the high-intensity treatment, but packages of time-limited therapy sessions are offered and reviewed frequently.

Nationally, one in two people receiving therapies through IAPT services recover and one in three show significant improvement in their mental health (NHS, 2018). IAPT services are also building on existing services to ensure that people with long-term physical conditions and medically unexplained symptoms (MUS) receive evidence-based psychological treatments. Evidence suggests that 40% of people with depression and anxiety disorders also have a long-term physical condition, and 30% of people with long-term physical conditions and 70% with MUS also have mental health conditions (NHS, 2018). Therefore, these services aim to ensure that people with long-term physical conditions and MUS have the same access to NICE-recommended psychological therapies as other people. Mental health and physical health services are coordinated to work together with the patient to ensure that they achieve the best outcome for the patient (Department of Health, 2011a).

The problems indicated above have a direct cost to society and the NHS. Without the involvement of IAPT, people may have been on long waiting lists, taking inappropriate medication or even continuing to experience health problems that they were unable to understand, resulting in taking time off work.

As indicated earlier (see *Section 6.2.7 Computerised CBT*), people can access help on a variety of platforms. IAPT services offer not only the traditional face-to-face CBT, but also the computer-based format.

ACTIVITY 6.5

Think about how the varying costs that experiencing a mental health problem that is not being treated may impose on:
1. The individual
2. The family and friends of the individual
3. Society.

6.3.4 Crisis resolution and home treatment teams (CRHTTs)

A mental health crisis is a situation that requires immediate support, care and intervention from an urgent and emergency mental health service. Examples might be someone who is experiencing a psychotic episode, is self-harming or is suicidal. The distress and concern of others would be of such a degree that, without the CRHTT, the person would fit the criteria for acute inpatient admission.

The widespread introduction of crisis resolution teams began in 2000, but they have not been fully integrated into services nationally. Consequently, the NHS Long Term Plan (NHS, 2019) commits to a 24/7 community-based mental health crisis response for adults and older adults across England by 2020/2021. Such services are based on the premise that a crisis, by definition, will pass. However, without the necessary support it can lead to deterioration in quality of life or to reinforcement of existing coping strategies that may not be the most effective. The CRHTTs strive to address ineffective coping strategies by offering an alternative to acute inpatient admission with targeted, intensive home treatment in a time-sensitive way.

6.3.5 Early intervention services (EIS)

Early intervention services were developed to support and treat people aged between 14 and 35 years. However, NICE has suggested that the service should be for all ages (NHS England, NCCMH and NICE, 2016). Most commonly the early intervention team (EIT) becomes involved with people who are experiencing a psychotic episode, and this may be their first experience of such an episode. Many of the people receiving help will continue to experience difficulties and often EITs augment what has become traditional psychological services (CBT and talking therapies, with the option of medication) with a recovery focus.

The EIT is generally multidisciplinary, with doctors, psychologists, nurses, social workers and support workers, all working together at an individual level. An EIT was found to be better than traditional mental health services at maintaining contact with patients and at reducing hospital readmissions (Craig *et al.*, 2004). Another study found that the introduction of EIS increased functional recovery rates at two years from around 15% to over 50% (Fowler *et al.*, 2009).

6.3.6 Mental health liaison

Mental health liaison services are opportunely based in A&E departments of general hospitals. Here they are best placed to respond to the needs of people with mental health problems, who are three times more likely than people without a mental health problem to attend A&E and five times more likely to be admitted to a general hospital as an emergency (Dorning, Davies and Blunt, 2015). The primary task of mental health liaison is to identify, assess and respond to mental health crises in the A&E department. This may also extend to other areas in the general hospital, such as medical assessment units, maternity services and step-down services from high dependency. Mental health liaison services have a remit to treat the associated symptoms and provide the patient with ongoing support, but they often work beyond this, through education and support of colleagues within the general hospital.

The NHS Long Term Plan (NHS, 2019) states that acute hospitals will have an all-age mental health liaison service in A&E departments and inpatient wards by 2020/2021. It is intended that 50% of these services will meet the 'core 24' standard of providing 24-hour care seven days a week, with a distinct team based in the hospital providing mental health care in a physical health setting. By 2023/2024, it is envisaged that 70% of liaison services will meet this standard, with a view to reaching the target of 100% thereafter.

6.3.7 Forensic services

In 1843 Daniel McNaughton killed Private Secretary Edward Drummond in a failed attempt to assassinate the British Prime Minister. This pivotal incident led to the establishment of the McNaughton Rules, under which the perpetrator of a crime is found not guilty by reason of insanity. This defence rests on the premise that a crime comprises mental and physical aspects. *Mens rea* refers to having an understanding that a specific act constitutes a crime and *actus reus* is the physical act itself (Trebilcock and Weston, 2019). In the instance of Daniel McNaughton there was no debating the physical aspect, as he was seen by witnesses to perpetrate the act. However, he was found to have impaired mental health to such a degree that he lacked awareness that, in committing this act, he was perpetrating a crime. This is the basis on which we still judge whether someone can be held accountable for crimes today.

It can be tempting to assume that crimes, particularly ones that outrage society, must have been committed when someone was 'not in their right mind'. This enables us to gain some distance from the perpetrator, as such 'othering' can make us feel less disturbed by it. However, we know that the relationship between mental health problems, crime and violence is complicated. Someone who perpetrates a heinous act can be aware of its gravity, that it is a crime and do it anyway, thereby demonstrating *mens rea* and *actus reus* as discussed above. It is also the case that someone with a mental health problem is far more likely to harm themselves than another person, as consistently illustrated by the National Confidential Inquiry into Suicide and Safety in Mental Health (University of Manchester, 2018).

Forensic mental health services are based on the premise that a therapeutic rather than a custodial approach is required if a mental health problem has had such a profound impact that an individual cannot be held responsible for their actions. Someone in this situation would be processed through the usual legal system, but would have been subject to assessment and review in order to make a recommendation to the court with regard to mental state. In such a case, any action would be to access care and treatment for the person in an appropriate setting, rather than to focus on punishment. If the individual would have gone to prison, they would instead be admitted to a forensic mental health service, where treatment and rehabilitation underpinned by the Mental Health Act 1983 can be implemented.

It may also be the case that someone found guilty of a crime and sent to prison suffers deterioration in mental health that requires care and treatment while serving their sentence. Should this deterioration occur to such a degree that the usual health care facility in the prison cannot provide the specialist intervention required, the person might be transferred to forensic mental health services. Once recovered, the person would then be conveyed back to prison to complete their sentence.

The umbrella term 'forensic mental health service' covers health care within prison, high, medium and low secure inpatient facilities, and a range of community services that support rehabilitation and recovery.

In England and Wales there are three high secure hospitals – Ashworth, Broadmoor and Rampton – providing around 700 beds, and approximately 60 medium secure units with 3500 beds (65% of these are within the NHS, the remainder are provided by the independent sector). Scotland has its own high secure provision, which also covers Northern Ireland – the State Hospital Scotland Carstairs, with 140 high secure beds.

The nature of this work means that assessment is crucial, both before any court action to ensure an appropriate outcome, and as an ongoing process. Assessment has a focus on therapeutic intervention, but undeniably must also take account of the need to protect the safety of the public while supporting people in their rehabilitation. Care and treatment in forensic mental health services is an interprofessional pursuit undertaken by a range of professionals, including nurses, social workers, occupational therapists, doctors, psychologists, pharmacists and support workers.

6.3.8 Recovery services

Recovery services focus on mental health and wellbeing and have an ethos that aims for, in lay language, recovery (resumption of functioning as it was before an illness, e.g. recovery following a broken leg). However, recovery services accept that recovery in the lay sense may not be achieved by all who are involved in the service. An episode of mental ill health can have long-term effects on an individual and can change the goals and aspirations they held before they became ill.

The focus of recovery services is to build resilience and self-esteem, while also and importantly refocusing goals to achievable ones in the individual's control. Crucially, recovery is not solely focused on symptom removal; rather, it focuses on coping and development of skills to manage any symptoms.

The Mental Health Foundation (2019) describes recovery as a process that can be understood using the acronym CHIME (Connectedness, Hope and optimism, Identity, Meaning and purpose, Empowerment). For recovery, the most important element in this process is the highlighting of hope and self-identity. Commonly, mental ill health is seen as a lifelong debilitating and isolating illness that stigmatises views and aspirations of all. CHIME indicates a pathway to a purposeful life where people who have experienced mental ill health resume work, studies and family life. Recovery services commonly work with families, friends and other service providers to facilitate a person's inclusion in everyday life. Such an approach to providing care involves a joint aim across all those involved.

6.4 Roles

6.4.1 Mental health nurses

A mental health nurse and a community mental health nurse have very similar roles, and they are both registered mental health nurses. However, the mental health nurse works in inpatient mental health settings and the community nurse works with patients who mainly live independently in the community. Whether they work in an inpatient setting or in the community, both provide care to people with mental health conditions. Mental health nurses provide a range of interventions to support people to recover and stay well, which may include short-term crisis intervention or longer-term support and treatment. Mental health nurses work with and support people who have a wide range of mental health conditions, such as anxiety, depression, schizophrenia and bipolar disorder. They also may specialise in working with a particular group, for example in forensic mental health services.

A mental health nurse may also act as a care coordinator, the person who coordinates and monitors care provided to people with mental health conditions (care coordination can be provided by other professionals as well, such as occupational therapists or social workers) (Goodwin and Lawton-Smith, 2010). An individual's care coordinator is not necessarily the person who provides all of their care; they will work with other health professionals to assess the individual's needs and coordinate the care that is required, which may be via another professional or team. The care that the individual requires will be written into a care plan by their coordinator and this will set out how professionals and other services will meet their needs. The care plan will be regularly reviewed to check the individual's progress (see *Section 6.2.1*).

6.4.2 Consultant psychiatrists

Consultant psychiatrists are health professionals who are medically qualified to diagnose illness, manage treatment and provide a range of therapies for complex and serious mental illness. This is a clinical role that involves the prescribing of medication, clinical leadership via supervision, accountability for patient care, providing consultant opinion on complex clinical problems, and diagnosis, prevention and treatment of mental disorders. Consultant psychiatrists are involved in the assessment and detention of patients under the Mental Health Act 1983. They generally work as part of a multidisciplinary team in order to assess, treat and prevent further deterioration in a mental health condition. Psychiatrists may specialise in certain areas, such as forensic or paediatric psychiatry, teaching and training innovation, and research (RCPsych, 2010).

6.4.3 Graduate mental health workers

Most people experiencing mental health difficulties will be supported in primary care services such as GP practices. To ensure the right mix of skill and expertise within the NHS, a need was identified for practitioners who could promote good mental health, offer support through therapeutic interventions and signpost to other services. This led to the establishment of primary care graduate mental health workers (also called psychological wellbeing practitioners). Further information on the role can be found at: nationalcareers.service.gov.uk/job-profiles/primary-care-graduate-mental-health-worker.

Since the introduction of graduate mental health workers in the early 2000s, the need for their services has not diminished: the NHS Long Term Plan (NHS, 2019) states that nine out of ten adults with mental health problems are supported in primary care and that half of all mental health problems are established by the age of 14, with three-quarters established by 24 years of age. It is therefore crucial that timely intervention is available and accessible. This links to Making Every Contact Count (PHE, 2018a), given that the vast majority of the population will engage with primary care services of some kind throughout their lifetime, which is why mental health is a crucial part of primary care.

6.4.4 Psychodynamic psychotherapists

Psychodynamic psychotherapy focuses on the unconscious patterns of the person's inner world through the relationship with the therapist, who is able to interpret these and help make sense of them (see *Sections 2.6* and *6.2.4*). This requires the psychotherapist to have engaged in rigorous clinical training, their own personal therapy and ongoing clinical supervision. A therapist who has sufficient clinical training and expertise is often a member of and accredited by bodies such as the British Psychoanalytic Council (BPC), the UK Council for Psychotherapy (UKCP) and the Association of Child Psychotherapists (ACP). These bodies help to ensure that the models and approaches used by therapists are robust and suitable for the person's individual needs.

Psychodynamic psychotherapists also work with groups, teams and organisations. Psychodynamic psychotherapy is a transferable approach that enables the therapist to work with other professionals in whatever environment they are needed. One example was the work of Isabel Menzies Lyth, who spent time observing nurses in a teaching hospital and was able to make sense of how the nurses managed their reactions to the difficult aspects of nursing, such as death and dying, life-changing injuries and loss of functioning. These, she said, were not really managed at all, and instead the nurses dispelled the associated anxiety by using sophisticated and unconscious defence mechanisms. These included maintaining a distance between the nurse and patient, such as referring to them by their condition rather than their name. The often unspoken but shared expectation that patients would wear night clothes rather than their usual attire served to diminish individuality. Other organisational rituals might include ensuring that everyone is washed before breakfast, despite there being no evidence-based rationale for this; such a ritual then becomes more important than promoting choice and individualised care.

Menzies Lyth also observed the impact on nurses themselves, such as an increase in sickness rates, a decrease in morale and student nurses leaving for reasons other than course failure. It may be surprising to learn that this work by Menzies Lyth was undertaken in the 1950s, given that it has clear relevance today. The way to avoid the use of defence mechanisms in the way that Menzies Lyth (1959) described is to provide an open and supportive organisational culture where the stresses, strains and emotional labour of nursing can be talked about and support offered.

Thus, psychodynamic psychotherapy can be valuable not only as a therapeutic intervention, but also in relation to organisations as a whole. It can aid understanding of what is really going on in a team – if this can be talked about, defence mechanisms can be understood and alternatives that take realistic account of the challenges can be introduced and supported.

ACTIVITY 6.6

Reflect on your personal and observed experiences of how anxiety may be managed in clinical practice. Have you ever distanced yourself to make the work more bearable? Do you see others doing this too?

6.4.5 Support workers

The support worker role in health care has had various titles such as nursing assistant, health care assistant and nursing auxiliary. In the past the role was aimed at supporting more senior staff in completing their duties and carrying out the 'less glamorous' roles of health care.

The Centre for Mental Health (2017) reported on the development of the role and the need for it in mental health multidisciplinary teams. Since then the role has started to evolve into a more autonomous position requiring an increased level of skills and knowledge. In mental health the role has developed most clearly in community settings, where support workers have their own clients and are responsible for maintaining and compiling reports, assessing client needs and developing care plans. Much of their work is conducted independently and requires a proactive approach to health care.

The support worker role demands particular skill and knowledge related to engagement and communication with, commonly, individuals with more complex problems, who are difficult to engage.

Although the role was rather limited by further workforce developments (e.g. the role of the nursing associate), numbers of support workers are still rising (NHS Digital, 2021) and the role is consolidating around specific areas, such as employment support work and peer support work. Despite this consolidation, many support workers continue to work in a range of teams and have embraced a developing role with an increasing level of complexity and responsibility.

6.4.6 Approved mental health professionals (AMHPs)

These may be social workers, nurses, occupational therapists and psychologists who have undergone specific preparation in order to carry out duties under the Mental Health Act 1983. Primarily these duties focus on the coordination of assessment and admission to hospital when a section of the Mental Health Act is deemed to be required (Department of Health, 2015). Following two medical recommendations, the AMHP will decide whether or not to make an application for the detention of the person. This requires sound legal knowledge of the Mental Capacity Act 2005, including Liberty Protection Safeguards and alternatives to admission (see *Section 8.2*). The AMHP must ensure that the patient and their nearest relative are involved (CQC, 2018). The AMHP must ensure that the person's rights and dignity are upheld, in conjunction with the legal responsibilities inherent in supporting actions that are in the best interests of the person.

CHAPTER SUMMARY

Key points to take away from *Chapter 6*:
- ☑ Mental health work requires an in-depth awareness and knowledge of both physical and psychological theory, and also of the biochemical working of drugs and neuroprocessing.
- ☑ Self-help materials can broaden the opportunity for people to access help from non-statutory NHS services, at a time convenient to them and in a format of their choice: telephone, computerised, from manuals, etc.
- ☑ The roles in mental health care, including nursing roles, are continually evolving and often have links with and governance from other professional bodies (e.g. the British Psychological Society).
- ☑ Specialist teams (e.g. IAPT) have demonstrated the effectiveness of time-limited interventions with structured aims that adult health care practitioners can refer patients to.

Questions

Question 6.1	Detail the things that are needed to develop a therapeutic relationship with a person experiencing mental health difficulties. *(Learning outcome 6.1)*
Question 6.2	List and then describe some of the roles of professionals involved in mental health care. *(Learning outcome 6.2)*
Question 6.3	Describe the links between mental and physical health and the role of the health care practitioner. *(Learning outcomes 6.3 and 6.4)*
Question 6.4	Describe the range of health care provisions available to practitioners and people with mental health difficulties. *(Learning outcome 6.5)*

FURTHER READING

Gilburt, H., Peck, E., Ashton, B., Edwards, N. and Naylor, C. (2014) *Service Transformation: the lessons learned from mental health.* King's Fund. Available at: www.kingsfund.org.uk/sites/default/files/field/field_publication_file/service-transformation-lessons-mental-health-4-feb-2014.pdf (accessed 23 June 2021).

NHS England, National Collaborating Centre for Mental Health and National Institute for Health and Care Excellence (2016) *Achieving Better Access to 24/7 Urgent and Emergency Mental Health Care Part 2.* Available at: www.england.nhs.uk/wp-content/uploads/2016/11/lmhs-guidance.pdf (accessed 23 June 2021).

Parry, S. (ed.) (2019) *Handbook of Brief Therapies: a practical guide.* SAGE Publications.

Wright, K.M. and McKeown, M. (eds) (2018) *Essentials of Mental Health Nursing.* SAGE Publications.

ONLINE RESOURCES

British National Formulary (BNF): https://bnf.nice.org.uk/

Mental health apps: www.nhs.uk/apps-library/category/mental-health

Talking therapies: www.mentalhealth.org.uk/a-to-z/t/talking-therapies

Self-help therapies: www.nhs.uk/mental-health/talking-therapies-medicine-treatments/talking-therapies-and-counselling/self-help-therapies

Chapter 7
Mental health in later life

Rachel Price and Katie Davis

LEARNING OUTCOMES

By the end of this chapter you should be able to:

7.1 Identify the impact ageing has on mental health

7.2 Outline the most common mental health problems affecting older people

7.3 Understand service provision available for older people with mental health problems

7.4 Demonstrate an awareness of evidence-based interventions that can be adopted to support older people with mental health problems

7.5 Understand the complex relationship between physical and mental health in the ageing population.

7.1 Introduction

The mental health needs of older people can often be overlooked and accepted as just a normal part of the ageing process. Consequently, the promotion of positive mental health and investment in research have fallen behind in this area, as it is viewed as less of a priority than children or adults with mental health problems.

'Older age' is a difficult concept to define. As life expectancy continues to rise, people are living and working longer. Lifestyle and family relationships are different from those of past generations. However, developments in medicine and health care, created to meet these differences, have led to people living independently for longer.

The 'older person' has often been defined in terms of chronological age, with 65 as the threshold, and organisations, especially in mental health, often use the age of 65 as a criterion for accessing older people's services. Chronological age may determine service access, eligibility for retirement and associated benefits. However, it is important to consider the biological, psychological and social age of the individual to inform the delivery of person-centred care.

Although life expectancy is growing for the ageing population, older people are increasingly likely to be living with long-term health conditions, and a wide body of evidence shows that comorbid mental health problems and long-term conditions in the older person lead to significantly poorer health outcomes, poorer quality of life, increased risk of premature death and a higher utilisation of acute NHS care (Stafford *et al.*, 2018).

It is important to recognise that the symptoms of mental illness in older people can be very different from those experienced by younger people. This may be attributed to the prevalence of comorbid physical health conditions (see *Figure 7.1*), as older people with such comorbidities are more likely to develop a mental disorder (RCPsych, 2019).

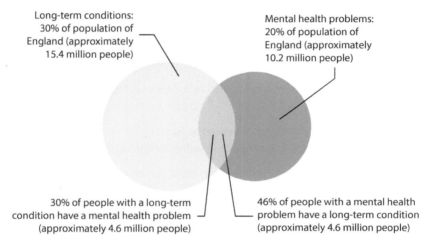

Long-term conditions: 30% of population of England (approximately 15.4 million people)

Mental health problems: 20% of population of England (approximately 10.2 million people)

30% of people with a long-term condition have a mental health problem (approximately 4.6 million people)

46% of people with a mental health problem have a long-term condition (approximately 4.6 million people)

Figure 7.1 *The overlap between long-term conditions and mental health problems (Naylor et al., 2012). Reproduced with permission from the King's Fund and Centre for Mental Health.*

Evidence highlights that mental health services for people over the age of 65 are underfunded and that government policy has paid little attention to the complex needs of older people; the discrimination that older people face arises not only in wider society but also within health and social care organisations (RCPsych, 2018). With this in mind, it is important that the nursing community is understanding, informed and prepared to address the complex needs of the older person, particularly if they are experiencing mental ill health.

Understanding the mental health conditions experienced by the older person is increasingly important for all fields of nursing practice. The publication of the Francis Report (Mid Staffordshire NHS Foundation Trust, 2013) and subsequent response by the Nursing and Midwifery Council (NMC, 2013) has demonstrated a need for nursing staff to be well trained and better prepared to support the complex needs of older vulnerable people. This chapter will explore the most common mental health problems experienced by the ageing population and will also examine resources and interventions available to support the management of older people's mental health in order to enhance healthy ageing.

ACTIVITY 7.1

Think about factors that support healthy ageing, and make a list of all the elements that you think will support people to age well and maintain quality of life. Make a list of what you think the consequences will be if an older person is not able to maintain activities of daily living or remain physically and mentally 'well'.

7.2 **The mental health of older people**

The onset of mental health conditions can occur at any point in life. However, older people can experience additional stressors that are more closely associated with ageing. For example, older people are more likely to experience a decline in function and ability to maintain activities of daily living, loss of mobility, increased chronic pain, frailty and comorbid physical health conditions. They are also more likely to experience a reduction in socio-economic status, poverty, psychological distress, bereavement, isolation and loneliness. These factors can have an impact on their mental health and wellbeing to varying degrees.

Changes in the cognitive function of older people can also indicate the onset of mental illness and these changes are associated with change and structural decline in the composition of the brain.

Mental health conditions experienced by older people can have three distinct explanations:
1. They are long-term mental health problems that arose in childhood and/or adult life and continue to affect the individual as they age.
2. They are new-onset mental health problems arising from psychosocial challenges and a change in physical health.
3. They result from the onset of cognitive change caused by organic brain changes due to neurological disease or organic brain disease.

ACTIVITY 7.2

Think about your own experiences of caring for someone or simply knowing someone with a mental health problem in later life. What type of mental illness has this person experienced? Are you able to identify whether this mental illness has arisen through psychosocial or physical health challenges, or because of organic or neurological brain changes? What type of conditions have you come across?

7.3 **Mental health conditions in older age**

It is estimated that 40% of older people registered with a GP have a mental health condition; this rises to 50% of older people who are being treated in an acute general hospital and 60% of older people who are residing in a residential care home or nursing home (Age UK, 2019).

It is important to recognise that changes in the mental health and wellbeing of older people are not just about 'old age' or 'getting old'. Adopting such perspectives means that the welfare and mental health of the older person may be neglected, causing a significant impact on quality of life. It is therefore imperative that the mental health of older people is given as much investment and care as their physical health.

Older people are entitled to a mental health assessment and treatment as much as any other age group. It is therefore important for all front-line staff to be aware of the main mental health conditions and their symptoms experienced by older people, so that the right intervention can be delivered in a timely manner.

7.3.1 Mood disorders in later life

Mood disorders experienced by older people are clinically significant, as the onset of depression in particular has the potential to have a substantial impact on quality of life and global function. There remains a persistent challenge in seeing the symptoms of depression as something other than a symptom of ageing and not something inevitable that there is little opportunity to resolve.

Although stress, loss and physical comorbidities are common in older people, the debilitating symptoms of depression should not be accepted as a routine part of growing older. The challenge that may face the health care specialist is that the common symptoms associated with depression, such as low mood, sleep disturbance, loss of appetite, feelings of guilt and hopelessness, social withdrawal, slowed thinking and cognitive change, may present in a more subtle or atypical way in an older person.

The interaction of mood disorders with physical health comorbidities may also confuse the picture, particularly when the signs and symptoms of a depressive episode are attributable to a physical illness or to a psychological reaction to physical disease and illness.

Depression

Changes in mood and the onset of depression in an older person should be viewed as a mental health condition that can be treated effectively and simultaneously alongside any existing physical health comorbidity. Effective recognition of depressive syndromes is a prerequisite for the introduction of effective treatment, yet the identification of mood disorders in older people is often overlooked.

For general nurses working in hospital or community settings there is an opportunity for the early identification of depression and other mood disorders, and these need emphasising alongside any physical health symptoms and functional disability. It is important to acknowledge that as a general nurse you may be the first professional to become involved with the individual; being aware of mood changes that typically affect older people will facilitate more effective signposting and the potential to improve health and quality of life outcomes.

ACTIVITY 7.3: CLINICAL CASE STUDY – LINA

Lina is a 75-year-old woman who has an appointment at her local GP practice. The usual GP is on holiday, so Lina sees the locum GP, who reviews her notes prior to the appointment. The locum reads that Lina has attended the practice four times in the past seven weeks, complaining of weight loss, poor appetite, decreased energy and finding it difficult to get to sleep.

At her appointment Lina complains that her symptoms are getting worse and that she is now struggling to go out and do her shopping, meet with friends and go to her art class; the locum GP identifies a further 2.75 kg loss in weight since her last attendance three weeks ago.

In Lina's notes her own GP has noted that, if she returns to the surgery with no resolution of symptoms, he plans to refer her to the gastroenterology outpatient team for a review.

The locum GP asks Lina about her mood and if anything is worrying her and Lina explains that two months ago her dog died and since then she has felt upset. Lina says she feels 'silly' about getting upset, especially as it was her husband's dog, but it was the only company she had since her husband died 12 months ago. Lina becomes very distressed during the conversation and tells the locum GP that she feels she 'no longer has anything to live for' and 'part of me knows this is silly, it was only a dog, but I can't seem to get over it'.

What do you think may be happening to Lina? Do you think a gastroenterology appointment should be requested as a priority? What other options should be considered?

The risk factors associated with the onset of depression in older people are often complex. However, studies have identified several factors that can increase the risk (Cahoon, 2012; NHS England, 2017):

- chronic physical health problems (including pain)
- polypharmacy
- bereavement
- functional decline, both physical and mental
- social isolation
- substance use/misuse/dependency
- family or personal history of depression.

In addition to these risk factors, certain populations are classed as being at higher risk of experiencing depression in later life:

- women
- individuals experiencing some form of sleep disorder.

The classic symptoms of depression in older people are similar to those experienced by adults and younger people, but biological and physical symptoms may be more prevalent. It is important to recognise that an older person may deny feelings of sadness or low mood but describe symptoms such as weight loss, insomnia, slowed movement and pain. The person may also have developed some mild memory problems and possibly appear confused. Behaviour may become withdrawn or, conversely, the individual may frequently seek out the support of others to meet their needs. Depressive disorders can be classified as mild, moderate or severe, depending on the intensity of symptoms. It is also important to recognise that in more severe episodes the individual may experience symptoms of psychosis (WHO, 2019a).

There are several other mood disorders that older people may experience that are associated with a depressive type illness. For example, dysthymia is a chronic and less severe form of depression; the symptoms can alter in intensity, but they do not disappear completely and, for a diagnosis, must have persisted for at least two years. An older person faced with a specific life stressor that induces symptoms of low mood and depression (e.g. the death of a spouse or partner, moving into long-term care or receiving a life-limiting health diagnosis) may develop an adjustment disorder with depressed mood.

Bipolar disorder

Bipolar disorder is less prevalent among older people but it does account for 8–10% of acute psychiatric admissions, and the management and treatment of bipolar disorder remains a significant part of an old age psychiatrist's caseload (Rubinsztein, Sahakian and O'Brien, 2019). Bipolar disorder is characterised by two or more episodes in which the person's mood and activity levels are significantly disturbed; on some occasions this disturbance involves an elevation of mood with increased energy and activity (hypomania or mania) and on others a lowering of mood and reduced energy and activity (depression).

Older people with a diagnosis of existing or new-onset bipolar disorder are more likely to have a lower life expectancy than the general population. There is also an increased likelihood that an older person will have comorbid physical health problems such as type 2 diabetes, respiratory and cardiovascular conditions and other endocrine abnormalities, which may have arisen because of lifestyle, the condition itself or even the treatment for bipolar disorder (Rise, Haro and Gjervan, 2016). Most research into bipolar disorder has been conducted in adult populations aged 18–65, but there is clear evidence that a bipolar diagnosis in an older person is associated with increased cognitive decline, an increased use of polypharmacy and a higher reliance on informal support (Dautzenberg *et al.*, 2016).

7.3.2 Anxiety and related disorders in later life

Anxiety is a prevalent disorder in the older population and substantial numbers of older people experience an anxiety disorder with a comorbid depressive illness. Anxiety disorder in the older population is twice as common as dementia and four to six times more common than major depression. As a result, it is associated with higher mortality rates, contributes to the onset or heightening of disability, has a significant impact on quality of life and causes significant distress (Koychev and Ebmeier, 2016).

Diagnosing anxiety disorders in older people presents a significant challenge, as the symptoms often mimic physical health complaints. Shortness of breath, chest pain, palpitations, abdominal pain and digestive problems are common symptoms of anxiety, but can also feature in physical health conditions such as anaemia, cardiovascular and cerebrovascular disease, hyperthyroidism, diabetes and hypoglycaemia. This makes it important for an older person to have a full history of their symptoms recorded and to undergo physical health screening prior to making a diagnosis of anxiety, in order to exclude any acute or chronic physical health conditions. It is important to recognise that older people experiencing anxiety may present differently from younger people. People experiencing anxiety will often complain of worry, 'nerves', tension, tiredness and irritability; however, older people may report more somatic symptoms, such as pain, discomfort and palpitations, which potentially can be confused with the exacerbation or onset of a physical health condition. This may explain why anxiety is often unrecognised and undertreated in the older population.

Generalised anxiety disorder (GAD) is the most common form of anxiety experienced by older people. It is associated with the onset of excessive worrying that is difficult to control and may be related to specific life events or activities. These symptoms need to have been present for over six months and are often accompanied by sleep disturbance, changes in mood and somatic symptoms.

7.3.3 Psychosis in later life

The onset of psychosis in older people is very challenging, as there is more likely to be a secondary reason for the condition's onset compared with psychosis presenting in younger people.

The symptoms of psychosis have been described in *Chapter 4*. Psychosis with onset in older age is likely to be less severe than psychosis in younger adults, and late-onset psychotic symptoms have been linked to neurological change associated with underlying organic brain disease. Older people who live alone, who are socially isolated or have sensory problems, especially hearing loss, are more likely to experience psychotic symptoms, and it is essential that assessment of an older person presenting with psychotic symptoms should include a comprehensive biopsychosocial assessment to ensure that these factors are identified.

The onset of schizophrenia in older age is associated with a higher incidence of delusions and visual, tactile and olfactory hallucinations that are more clinically evident; yet older people are less likely than younger people to experience negative symptoms of schizophrenia, such as depression, apathy and poor motivation. Psychotic symptoms may occur in older people because of other clinical conditions, not just schizophrenia. Conditions such as dementia, psychotic depression, delirium and substance misuse can all play a part in the onset of psychosis and this demonstrates the importance of identifying the underlying condition.

Delirium and psychosis due to substance misuse are transient and can be managed clinically when the underlying cause is resolved.

Psychotic depression requires specialist management from older people's mental health services to ensure that appropriate treatment and support are available to potentially resolve the condition. Psychosis that arises in dementia is much more challenging to manage, as dementia is a progressive disease for which there is no cure; yet with specialist support from older people's mental health services symptoms can potentially be reduced and managed more effectively.

7.3.4 Bereavement in later life and mental health

Bereavement is the experience of having encountered a loss and it is defined as fundamentally an emotional, behavioural, biological and cognitive process (Ryan and Coughlan, 2011). Although loss can be experienced at any age, there are distinctive challenges that the older person may face. Older people are more likely to experience loss and bereavement than any other age group. Death is more widely associated with ageing, disability, declining physical health and frailty, which are factors more commonly experienced in the older population.

A normal grief reaction has been described as having five key stages: denial, anger, bargaining, depression and acceptance (Kubler-Ross and Kessler, 2005). Although depression is suggested to be a key part of the grieving process, this stage is different from the condition that has previously been explored in this chapter, which is classed as a clinical depressive illness. In grief, the experience of depression relates to a normal phase in which the nervous system temporarily shuts down in response to the emotional upheaval that bereavement induces; this will resolve and is a normal part of the grieving process. It is important to recognise that each individual's experience of grief is unique and although we should understand the stages of grief that can be encountered, we should not expect a person to respond in a way we think should be typical.

Within the older age group, it is also more common for individuals to experience a sense of loss and a bereavement reaction not only to a death but also to significant life change, such as a move from independent living into a care home, a spouse who has developed a life-limiting or debilitating illness or the onset of the person's own complex physical health challenges. It is important to recognise that some older people are in fact resilient to bereavement and after the initial grieving period can adjust psychologically to the loss. Their reaction to a bereavement will depend on what resources they have available to them. Older people with a good social support network, financial stability and stable mental health prior to the bereavement are less likely to experience a complicated grief reaction. For older people experiencing a bereavement without these protective factors there is an increased risk that an abnormal grief reaction will occur and an increased likelihood that a significant depressive episode will develop.

The challenge for nurses caring for older people who are recently bereaved is to identify whether their reaction to the loss suggests a normal grief reaction. This is particularly important because older people are more likely to develop symptoms of clinical depression following a bereavement that, if left untreated, can cause significant mental health problems (Ryan and Coughlan, 2011).

ACTIVITY 7.4: CLINICAL CASE STUDY – MAX

Max is 78 years of age and was admitted to hospital following a hip fracture nine days ago. He had fallen down the stairs rushing to open the door for the paramedics, who were attending for his wife after he found her in bed unresponsive. Max was told in A&E that his wife had died when he was on his way for an X-ray on his hip. Yesterday was her funeral.

The mental health liaison service has been called by the orthopaedic team to assess Max, as they feel he is depressed and needs to start antidepressants as soon as possible. The ward staff report that he is not reaching his recovery goals as anticipated and feel this is because he is depressed.

The mental health practitioner meets with Max and her handover to the orthopaedic ward team is that she would not recommend that Max starts antidepressants and that he will be offered a routine follow-up appointment by mental health services in eight weeks' time.

Why do you think the mental health practitioner did not advocate for antidepressant therapy to be prescribed? Why was the appointment for a mental health review arranged for eight weeks' time? Knowing the bereavement Max has experienced, what would be useful to consider when planning his care and supporting him to reach his recovery goals?

7.3.5 Alcohol and substance disorders in later life

Alcohol and substance misuse in older people are often overlooked because older adults are more likely to hide their dependency and less likely to seek the help of health care professionals. It is also important to recognise that the increased isolation of older people means that family and friends are not as involved in their day-to-day life and therefore alcohol and substance dependency issues often go largely unrecognised. The presence of comorbid physical health problems and polypharmacy can also often mask the symptoms of alcohol and substance dependency.

An older person may turn to alcohol and substance use as a way of managing their social isolation, as a coping strategy for bereavement, because of life stress and as a way of managing symptoms of physical health conditions. The use of substances and alcohol may also be because of lifelong behaviour that has continued into later life. Physiological changes associated with the ageing process make older people more vulnerable to the effects of consumption: for example, blood alcohol concentrations are likely to be higher for longer than in younger people and the effects of substance misuse on existing mental and physical health conditions may be greater. Add in the presence of comorbid physical and mental health conditions and prescribed medications and it is unsurprising that an older person with an alcohol or substance dependency problem is at higher risk of experiencing significant health complications and increased risk of hospitalisation, disability and even death.

Older people with mental health conditions are more likely to have alcohol and substance dependency problems, yet there is a lack of service provision for them and, as a result, they may present to services and organisations that have limited knowledge about the complex needs of older people. Older people presenting with complex substance and alcohol dependency issues should be referred to older people's mental health services for a full assessment of their needs if there is evidence of a comorbid mental health problem, or a referral should be made to specialist alcohol and substance misuse services if a primary mental disorder is not present.

7.3.6 Dementia

Dementia is not a normal part of the ageing process, is not an inevitable consequence of getting older and should not be viewed as a condition exclusively experienced by old people, particularly as one in 750 people diagnosed with dementia is under the age of 65. The number of people in the UK living with dementia is estimated to be around 850,000 and this is set to rise to around one million by 2025 (Prince *et al.*, 2014). Given the ageing population, developments in medical technology and increases in life expectancy this may be a conservative prediction. It is estimated that 25% of acute hospital beds are occupied by people with dementia and hospital stays are often longer and the discharge process more challenging because of the complex health and social care needs associated with this progressive disease. In a community setting people with dementia are often cared for by family members and informal carers, and estimates suggest around 700,000 people in the UK provide unpaid care for people with dementia, with almost half of these carers having their own disability or long-term illness (Prince *et al.*, 2014).

Dementia is a term that is used to describe a large and varied range of symptoms that arise when the structure of or cell composition of the brain are irreparably damaged. These symptoms may include a progressive decline in perception, reasoning, communication and memory. In addition there is a pervasive decline in the person's ability to undertake activities of daily living and carry out tasks and activities to maintain independence. There may also be marked changes in personality and behaviour. There are over 100 different types of dementia, but the most common are *Alzheimer's disease, vascular dementia, frontotemporal dementia* and *dementia with Lewy bodies*.

The Alzheimer's Society (www.alzheimers.org.uk) is a good resource for information on dementia. It has produced a series of publications and fact sheets that will not only improve your own knowledge of dementia and its different types but are also an excellent resource for people with dementia and their relatives who come into your care and require more information.

People with dementia face many challenges when accessing health care. These may include not having their rights for equality, inclusion and non-discrimination addressed. Tom Kitwood, in his seminal book on dementia care, *Dementia Reconsidered: the person comes first*, introduces the concept of malignant social psychology (Kitwood, 1997). This concept is based on the idea that individuals engage in behaviours that serve to undermine the wellbeing and personhood of the person with dementia (see *Table 7.1*). Person-centred care underpins contemporary

Table 7.1 *Kitwood's concept of malignant social psychology in relation to dementia (Kitwood, 1997)*

Malignancy concept	Definition
Treachery	The use of deception to distract or manipulate behaviour.
Disempowerment	Not allowing or enabling a person to use the abilities they still have.
Infantilisation	Treating the person like a child.
Intimidation	Causing the person to feel fearful as a result of threat or physical power.
Labelling	Using inappropriate terminology to refer to the person, for example 'demented', 'mentally infirm'.
Stigmatisation	Treating the person as if they were an outcast or that they serve no purpose.
Outpacing	Providing information or choices too quickly, thus making information difficult to understand.
Invalidation	Not acknowledging that the individual is still a person in their own right.
Banishment	Excluding the person either physically or emotionally.
Objectification	Treating the person as an object during self-care.
Ignoring	Conversing with others in the presence of the person and behaving as though they are not there.
Imposition	Forcing the person to do something.
Withholding	Failing to meet a need or not providing attention.
Accusation	Blaming the person for misunderstanding or lack of ability.
Disruption	Suddenly disturbing the person, interrupting their thoughts or activity.
Mockery	Making fun or making a joke at the expense of the person.
Disparagement	Telling the person that they are worthless or useless.

nursing practice, and viewing a person with dementia as more than the sum of a dementia diagnosis will serve you in developing an effective and therapeutic relationship. As the dementia progresses and the symptoms become more challenging for the person with the condition, it becomes more difficult to see that person behind all the complex behaviours associated with declining cognitive function. The loss of mental capacity, language and communication, social function and ability to maintain activities of daily living should not determine that the person is 'lost' or 'no longer there'. In fact, as health care professionals it is our duty and responsibility to ensure that the identity and the 'personhood' of the patient are maintained indefinitely.

Positive person-centred care that includes behavioural interventions is more successful in supporting people with dementia who present with behaviours that challenge. This is particularly useful knowledge for when a person with dementia is taken out of their most familiar environment, such as their own home, and admitted to an unfamiliar environment such as a hospital or care home.

7.3.7 Delirium

Delirium is not often characterised primarily as a mental illness. However, delirium is included in this chapter because it presents in half of people aged 70 and over who are admitted to hospital and its symptoms are often confused with chronic mental illness rather than recognised as a result of an underlying physical condition. The underlying acute physical condition triggers neuroinflammation, neurotransmitter imbalance and a chronic stress response, which prompt psychiatric symptoms.

Delirium can occur when a person experiences a physiological response to acute or chronic illness, after surgery, anaesthesia, trauma (especially following hip fracture), polypharmacy, if the person is dehydrated or constipated, or if the person has had episodes of delirium previously. The symptoms of delirium are often like those experienced by individuals who have a moderate to severe degree of dementia, and delirium is therefore often wrongly identified as a condition that requires mental health treatment as a priority.

It is essential that the underlying physical cause of the delirium is identified quickly. It is classed as a condition requiring **emergency assessment and management**, especially in older people, to improve mortality rates, to reduce admissions to long-term care, to reduce prolonged hospital admissions, to reduce the risk of the onset of dementia, and to improve quality of life.

Delirium is a testing condition for health care professionals because of the interplay between the underlying physical health causes and the occurrence of symptoms that present as the onset of a significant and challenging mental illness. Many health care environments where delirium presents have been offered little in the way of education and training in relation to its identification and management, and this factor contributes to the high mortality rate, especially among older people. Managing delirium can be challenging regardless of setting, as there are currently no medications approved for its treatment. It is therefore necessary to use non-pharmacological interventions to support the investigation and care of an older person with delirium.

Given the prevalence of delirium in all hospital and community-based care settings, it is essential that all front-line nursing staff are familiar with the common factors that precipitate its onset (see *Table 7.2*), are aware of the signs and symptoms of a delirium that has developed and are also skilled in delivering non-pharmacological interventions for older people with delirium.

Table 7.2 *Common factors that precipitate the onset of delirium (Fleet and Ernst, 2011)*

Common factors	Examples
Drugs	Alcohol or sedative withdrawal, hypnotics, opioids, antidepressants, recreational drug toxicity or withdrawal, corticosteroids, anticonvulsants.
Endocrine/metabolic	Thiamine deficiency, hypo-/hyperthyroidism, hypo-/hyperglycaemia, liver failure.
Environmental	Moving wards or a change in environment, loss of glasses or hearing aids, bright lighting, noise, sleep deprivation, catheters and treatment lines.
Fluid and electrolyte abnormality	Hypo-/hypernatraemia, hypercalcaemia, renal failure, dehydration.
Infections	Chest, urine, skin/ulcers, abdominal, central nervous system.
Neurological illness	Strokes, seizures, subdural haematoma.
Pain	Acute or chronic pain.
Respiratory/cardiovascular	Hypoxia, cardiac failure, myocardial infarction, organ/tissue ischaemia, hypercapnia.
Surgery	Orthopaedic, vascular/cardiac, gastrointestinal.
Urinary and faecal retention	Examination required; history is unreliable.

7.3.8 The three Ds in later life

The three most common mental health conditions experienced in later life are depression, dementia and delirium (the 'three Ds') and these conditions often overlap in terms of symptoms and presentation. The symptoms in some cases are so similar that it is very difficult to diagnose which of the three Ds has developed. The interplay between the conditions makes diagnosis challenging and that is why it is advisable for dementia not to be diagnosed in the older person if they are in an acute hospital or physically unstable, as delirium can often overlay dementia, making the clinical picture uncertain.

The main clinical symptoms associated with the three Ds are:
- memory problems
- low mood
- slowed thinking
- disturbed sleep
- fluctuating presentation
- changes in concentration
- agitation
- hallucinations and/or delusions.

Because of the similarities in presentation, the person may be prescribed treatment for depression, exposing them to potentially harmful side effects, when they are in fact experiencing a form of delirium that mimics a depressive illness. A clinical history is invaluable in supporting the diagnosis of dementia, delirium and/or depression, as both dementia and depression result in an insidious and progressive deterioration, whereas delirium arises in a matter of days or, in some cases, hours. *Table 7.3* outlines the prognosis and outcomes for the three conditions.

Table 7.3 *The three Ds: prognosis and outcomes*

Condition	Prognosis	If left untreated/undiagnosed
Depression	Treatable	Poor future treatment response. Longer recovery time. Increased risk of suicide/self-harm. Potential for onset of psychosis or serious depressive disorder.
Dementia	Progressive and life-limiting	Isolation. Reduced quality of life. Increased global risk to self. Lack of support. Lack of access to treatments and therapies. End of life care not coordinated.
Delirium	Treatable	Prolonged hospital stay/recurrent hospital admissions. Functional and cognitive decline. Increased mortality. Increased risk of requiring specialised care.

If an older person in hospital presents with symptoms of depression, dementia and/or delirium that are new in onset or are symptoms of an existing mental disorder a referral should be made to the mental health liaison service based in the hospital to ensure that an initial assessment and correct signposting are undertaken. For community-dwelling older people presenting with these symptoms, a referral to older people's mental health services is beneficial, to access specialist support from practitioners well versed in the identification and management of the three Ds.

7.4 Self-harm and suicide in later life

Some individuals experiencing mental health problems engage in self-harm, which is defined as an act or behaviour that causes injury or poisoning to themselves irrespective of the level of intent or level of medical significance. It is challenging to identify the prevalence of self-harm in older people, as the evidence relies heavily on individuals reporting that their actions were because of intentionally wanting to cause themselves harm. Individuals may feel less inclined to report self-harm because of feelings of shame or embarrassment, or because they are worried that they may be judged by others. It is important, especially in older people, that any incident involving self-harm is documented and the individual referred to a consultant psychiatrist as a matter of **urgency**. NICE guidance (NCCMH, 2012) notes that older people are more at risk of experiencing suicidal intent after an episode of self-harm, and this can be interpreted as an older person who has self-harmed being more likely to complete suicide compared with an older person with no history of self-harming behaviour. One of the most common reasons for older people self-harming is found to be related to a deterioration in physical health and loss of function. It is therefore important for older people with physical health problems to be routinely asked about how their physical health is affecting their mental health and wellbeing.

Mental illness is also a common factor influencing self-harm and completed suicide in older people: conditions such as severe depression, schizophrenia and psychosis, chronic anxiety, cognitive decline and substance misuse are all factors recognised as contributing to raising the risk of self-harm and suicide. Talking about self-harm and thoughts of suicide with older people does not encourage or increase the chances the individual will carry out an act of self-injury or increase suicidal tendencies. In fact, open discussions about self-harm and suicidal intent may reduce rather than increase the incidence. *Chapter 9* looks in more depth at risk and the principles set out in that chapter can be applied in the care of older people.

7.5 Mental health assessment in later life

Mental health assessment for older adults will follow a similar pathway to the assessment of adults under the age of 65. However, it is important to consider delirium first if symptoms have a rapid onset and are typical of the three Ds.

The building of a therapeutic relationship (see *Chapter 3*) will lay the foundation for a mental health assessment and allow for an open and honest conversation to take place.

There are various tools that can be used to aid the assessment of mental health in older people. Two of the most common are the MMSE and the GDS:

- The Mini-Mental State Examination (MMSE) is commonly used to assess cognitive function in older adults and is particularly useful to assess wherever someone has suspected dementia. It is not suitable for making a diagnosis but will give an idea of the person's orientation, short-term memory and language ability. The MMSE only takes around 10 minutes and is suitable for use in acute hospital environments and in the community.

- The 4-item Geriatric Depression Scale (GDS) is often used as a screening test for depression in older adults. It is quick and easy to use and consists of only four questions. It is suitable for use in primary care settings. However, it does have limited application in monitoring severe depression. The 15-item GDS can be used if time allows and to monitor ongoing depressive symptoms.

It should always be remembered that even if someone lives with one condition, it does not mean that other mental health problems should be ruled out. For example, if a person is living with dementia, it does not mean they cannot have depression as well.

ACTIVITY 7.5

Imagine you are assessing an older adult in a busy acute assessment unit. What are some of the potential barriers to assessment that you could encounter?

7.6 Therapeutic interventions in later life

Many therapeutic interventions suitable for the treatment of mental health problems in adults – for example, CBT – are also suitable for older adults. There are further treatments that might be considered specifically for older adults owing to the nature of their approach:

- *Reminiscence therapy* involves the sharing of memories, stories and life experiences. This can involve talking but also the use of objects to take someone back to an earlier experience in their life. Objects might include pictures, poems, clothes or uniforms, pieces of music, food and drink. Reminiscence therapy is often used with people with dementia but has also been shown to be effective with older people with depression (Alqam, 2018).

- *Music therapy* is used as an intervention across the life span, with children, adults and older adults. It has been shown to be particularly effective for people with dementia (Dowlen *et al.*, 2018). The video *Alive Inside* shows a powerful and emotive story of a man called Henry and the significant impact music has on his cognitive abilities. The video can be found at https://youtu.be/5FWn4JB2YLU.

- *Doll therapy* involves giving dolls to an older adult to hold, change or dress. Doll therapy is sometimes criticised for being condescending and for infantilising older people. However, it has been shown to reduce anxiety, improve communication and lessen distress in older adults, particularly those with dementia.

7.7 Pharmacological interventions in later life

Older adults are more likely to experience side effects and physical health problems from medication, so the rule is 'start low, go slow' when prescribing medication to older people (NHS England, 2017, p. 10).

NHS England (2017) advises that health care professionals should avoid prescribing the following medications to older adults:
- **Alpha-adrenoceptor blockers** (also known an alpha blockers). This type of medication is often used to treat high blood pressure and prostate problems. There is a suggested increased risk of dementia and delirium with these medications.
- **Antipsychotics**. These are used to treat symptoms of psychosis but can also be used to treat anxiety and some physical health problems. They are sometimes used when people with dementia present with agitation or challenging behaviour, but this is generally not recommended owing to increased risk of mortality.
- **Medication with a long half-life**. 'Half-life' means how long it takes for half of the dose to leave the bloodstream.

7.8 Mental health services for older people

The NHS Long Term Plan (NHS, 2019) highlights that there should be consistent access to mental health care for older adults and this should include access to psychological therapies, community services (including crisis services) and mental health liaison services within hospital settings.

In most areas of the UK, there will be specific community mental health teams that work with older adults. In hospital settings, older people with functional mental illness (such as depression, anxiety and psychosis) and those with dementia may be cared for in separate wards.

Many areas have further support for older adults through third-sector organisations such as Age UK and the Alzheimer's Society.

CASE STUDY 7.1: OPEN DOORS, SALFORD

Open Doors is funded and supported by Greater Manchester Mental Health NHS Foundation Trust (GMMH) and is described in its supporting literature as follows:

'The Open Doors Service is based on the promotion of living well with dementia and aims to literally "open doors" for people living with dementia, whose goals are to support the delivery, development and innovation of dementia services within Salford' (GMMH, 2018).

GMMH was the first NHS Trust in the UK to employ a person living with dementia in their services to truly ensure that a voice is given to people with the condition. The people living with dementia employed by GMMH are active in the Open Doors project as facilitators, and they help to support others with dementia and their care partners in Salford. Among the services developed by Open Doors are a dementia cafe, two support groups, a book club and a dining club. The project also takes an active part in research both within GMMH and with local universities.

CHAPTER SUMMARY

Key points to take away from *Chapter 7*:
- ☑ The mental health needs of older adults are often overlooked or dismissed.
- ☑ Depression is the most common mental health problem in older adults.
- ☑ Dementia, delirium and depression can present with similar symptoms in older adults and the conditions can often co-exist.
- ☑ Older adults are particularly vulnerable to side effects and increased mortality from medication.

Questions

Question 7.1	Consider the different ways ageing can affect mental health. *(Learning outcome 7.1)*
Question 7.2	Outline the most common mental health problems affecting older people and how they may present differently in older adults. *(Learning outcome 7.2)*
Question 7.3	Consider the service provision available for older people with mental health problems in your own Trust/area and the different ways they can be accessed. *(Learning outcome 7.3)*
Question 7.4	Consider the benefits and challenges of evidence-based interventions that can be adopted to support older people with mental health problems. *(Learning outcome 7.4)*
Question 7.5	Reflect on the complex relationship between physical and mental health in the ageing population and consider why mental health problems in older adults may sometimes be overlooked. *(Learning outcome 7.5)*

FURTHER READING

Age UK (2019) *Later Life in the United Kingdom*. Age UK.

Alzheimer's Society. www.alzheimers.org.uk

Isik, A.T. and Grossberg, G.T. (eds) (2019) *Delirium in Elderly Patients.* Springer.

National Institute for Health and Care Excellence (NICE) (2010) *Delirium: Prevention, Diagnosis and Management (clinical guideline CG103).* Available at: www.nice.org.uk/guidance/cg103 (accessed 23 June 2021).

Chapter 8
Legal and ethical issues

Will Hough and Elizabeth Garth

LEARNING OUTCOMES

By the end of this chapter you should be able to:

8.1 Develop an understanding of the legal frameworks used in mental health settings

8.2 Recognise the ethical theories and principles used in mental health care

8.3 Apply the legal frameworks and ethical principles to the examples given.

8.1 Introduction

What we are unable to see when out in practice are the internal thought processes that occur inside a nurse's head; we see the decisions made, without fully appreciating how they come to that decision. This chapter will outline the various legal frameworks mental health nurses are required to work within, as well as outlining the four ethical principles we are expected to uphold in any health care setting. We will discuss the application of the main ethical theories and how we may use these as the foundations for the decisions we make.

8.2 Legal frameworks

Legal frameworks are primary legislation passed as law which have gone through parliamentary processes. They are referred to as Acts or Statutes, which are made by government and passed into law to provide mandatory rules and regulations related to specific situations that everyone is required to follow. A failure to follow these would mean that we had committed an offence, making us liable to be prosecuted.

Statutes develop for different reasons. Sometimes it is recognised that some individuals or groups are poorly protected by the law; an example of this is the introduction of the Mental Capacity Act 2005, which protects people who do not have the capacity to make their own decisions. Legal frameworks can also be introduced to provide clearer direction within the law, as with the Equality Act 2010 (see *Section 8.2.1*). Whatever the purpose of a legal framework, all frameworks are relevant to all fields of nursing practice, as the NMC Code states that nurses, midwives and nursing associates must 'keep to the laws of the country in which you are practising' (NMC, 2018b, para. 20.4).

This section provides an overview of the commonly applied legal frameworks for mental health, considering their application in an adult health care setting. This section should be read alongside current UK government guidance, codes of practice and the details of each Act. Changes do occur; these are called amendments, and they can be intended to be permanent or temporary. An example of a temporary change is the Coronavirus Act 2020, which made amendments to the Mental Health Act. These amendments were in place from March 2020 to September 2020 to introduce ways of coping where staff shortages affected service availability. A permanent amendment is generally made in response to a review of the legislation, and the amendment then provides the standard we must work to.

8.2.1 Equality Act 2010

Legislation surrounding equality and preventing discrimination has been developing for more than half a century, with the introduction over this time of several pieces of legislation. These were brought together in 2010 by the UK government with the aims of harmonising and strengthening the law. The Act legally protects people from discrimination, including when receiving health care services. As a nurse it is important to have a good awareness of the protected characteristics identified by the Act, which are:

- age
- disability – for the purposes of the Act, a disability is defined as a physical or mental impairment that has substantial and long-term effects (lasting 12 months or more) on a person's ability to carry out normal day-to-day activities
- gender reassignment
- marriage and civil partnership
- race – for the purposes of the act, 'race' includes colour, nationality and ethnic or national origins
- religion or belief
- sex
- sexual orientation.

Under the Act you must not treat someone differently because of one of these protected characteristics. This includes making assumptions based on personal beliefs or a 'stereotype' about a characteristic instead of delivering individualised person-centred care. This can happen when someone holds a consciously judgemental viewpoint about a group, such as a racist viewpoint, and treats individuals from that group in a negative way, which is unacceptable in nursing.

There are also unconscious biases we need to be vigilant for within our practice. They can happen when we pick up small amounts of information about a group and form an idea about the needs and behaviours associated with the group based on a myth or inaccurate information. For example, if we think that dementia is common among older adults, we might assume that all older adults lack the capacity to make decisions. Another example would be a nurse on a medical ward whose knowledge of schizophrenia is limited to sensationalised press reporting about a specific incident. This has engendered in the nurse's thinking the incorrect belief that all people with that diagnosis are violent, which may negatively influence the way the nurse approaches a patient with a diagnosis of schizophrenia. The nurse may be cautious and limit contact to essential interactions such as medication rounds; the person is aware that the nurse is treating them differently from other patients and feels discriminated against.

When applying the Equality Act, clinical decisions must not be based on a suspicion related to experience, hearsay or unconscious bias and they must not deny an individual access to treatment because of one of the protected characteristics. This means, for example, not making assumptions about an individual's access to services based on a mental health diagnosis such as depression, or denying a service offered to others for reasons of a mental health diagnosis. Examples of this could be:
- disregarding physical health symptoms and making assumptions that tiredness, loss of appetite and weight loss were linked to an episode of depression, based on a patient's history of depression
- declining to visit a patient in their home when you would normally offer this community service, based on a diagnosis of schizophrenia, because of assumptions about the nature of the diagnosis.

Both of these are examples of discrimination against a person based on a disability.

8.2.2 Mental Capacity Act 2005 (as amended in 2018)

The Mental Capacity Act applies to people who are over the age of 16, and it was developed to protect people who do not have the capacity to make their own decisions. This is important when a nurse is considering and obtaining informed consent from an individual. To establish informed consent, you need to have assessed that the individual has capacity and has been provided with all the information they need to make the decision, and you must be satisfied that their consent is voluntary without coercion from any other person.

The assessment of capacity involves a two-stage test and the application of the five guiding principles. These decisions could include day-to-day decisions such as an inpatient making a choice of food or clothing, as well as life-changing decisions such as major surgery. The principles and the test support and guide those who care for people who may at that time be unable to make a decision for themselves.

The term 'person who lacks capacity' means a person who lacks capacity to make a particular decision or take a particular action for themselves at the time the decision or action needs to be taken. It does not mean that they will be unable to make every decision. For example, they may be able to decide what food to eat but be unable to comprehend and weigh up the information required to make a complex decision about a medical treatment.

The five statutory principles of the Mental Capacity Act are:

Principle 1 A person must be assumed to have capacity unless it is established that they lack capacity.

Principle 2 A person is not to be treated as unable to make a decision unless all practicable steps to help them to do so have been taken without success.

Principle 3 A person is not to be treated as unable to make a decision merely because they make an unwise decision.

Principle 4 An act done, or decision made, under this Act for or on behalf of a person who lacks capacity must be done, or made, in their best interests.

Principle 5 Before the act is done, or the decision is made, regard must be had to whether the purpose for which it is needed can be as effectively achieved in a way that is less restrictive of the person's rights and freedom of action.

The two-stage test is intended to help in the identification of individuals whose capacity may be impaired:

stage 1: determine the presence of an impairment of, or disturbance in the functioning of the mind or brain, and

stage 2: where an impairment or disturbance exists, determine whether this is preventing them from making the decision.

Stage 1 is the *diagnostic* part of the decision. It requires the evidence to be considered that may indicate an impairment or disturbance in functioning. An example could be an older person presenting with a head injury: it must be ascertained whether the impairment they show is diagnosed (e.g. dementia) or undiagnosed, and whether it is permanent (e.g. neurological damage) or temporary (e.g. alcohol intoxication), and consideration should be given to the urgency of the decision.

Stage 2 is the *functional test*. If any of the following indicators are present the person may *not* be able to make their own decision:

- lacking a general understanding of the decision that needs to be made, and why it needs to be made
- lacking a general understanding of the likely consequences of making or not making the decision
- being unable to understand, remember and use the information provided to them when making the decision
- being unable to, or unable to consistently, communicate the decision.

Any assessment of capacity must be appropriate to the job role and competency of the individual making the assessment. So, for example, a care assistant may assess the capacity of an individual to make a food choice, a district nurse the capacity to consent to changing of a dressing, a GP the capacity to understand and make a medication choice, etc. Where you do not have enough knowledge about the subject area of the decision you should refer to an appropriate professional to make the assessment, for example the mental health liaison team. The decision and the basis for the decision must be accurately recorded (NICE, 2020b), ideally in the patient's notes.

The decision to apply the Mental Capacity Act also needs to consider principle 5 before it is enacted:

> 'Before the act is done, or the decision is made, regard must be had to whether the purpose for which it is needed can be as effectively achieved in a way that is less restrictive of the person's rights and freedom of action.'

In deciding whether a person has capacity or not, there are suggested prompts in the guidance to help work through the decision-making process. These help us to think about the patient's needs and whether we have considered everything. It is important to adopt a person-centred approach and consider all factors that may be influencing a person's ability to make a decision. This will also help to gain an understanding of the best ways to support an individual in making a decision, and it will inform the process if this needs to move to a best interests decision (see *Section 8.2.1*). Nurses have an important role in this, as they are the professional most likely to have developed a therapeutic rapport with the individual. The prompts are as follows (adapted from NHS, 2021):

1. Does the person have all the information they need presented and communicated in a way they are able to understand? There are multiple mediums we can use to support us in providing information, including verbal, written, hearing and visual aids.
2. Could anyone else help with communication and support with decision-making, for example someone who knows the individual well such as a family member, friend or carer? In some circumstances professional support may be the best option and you may need to request an interpreter or an advocate.
3. Can the decision be delayed if they are likely to regain capacity? This needs to take into account individual factors, risks and presentation, for example alcohol or drug intoxication.
4. Consider whether there is a time of day when the person's understanding is better.
5. Are you in an environment where a person feels comfortable and able to discuss their decision? For example, is the area you are in private or are others able to overhear, which could inhibit engagement with decision-making? Is there a lot of noise, which may make it difficult for the person to hear information and concentrate to process it?
6. Have you allowed the person reasonable time to process the information and make a decision? For example, someone with depression may have the capacity to make a decision, but they may need more time to absorb information, ask questions and process the information.
7. Has the person got experience (or a lack of experience) in making health-related decisions? Knowing this may help you to understand the amount of information and support a person may need to make a decision.

8. Are there any concerns about the influence of others involving duress or coercion affecting the person's ability to make a decision?
9. Consider whether you are making an assumption based on age, appearance, condition and behaviour by objectively considering the information you have and the protected characteristics checklist in *Section 8.2.1*.

Most NHS Trusts have a Mental Capacity Act lead, who should be informed at the earliest opportunity where a decision has been made to apply the Mental Capacity Act and consider best interests.

Best interests decisions

Where an individual is assessed as not having capacity then principle 4 of the Mental Capacity Act must be applied. In an emergency setting or situation, owing to the urgency of the situation and potential risk to life, the assessment of capacity and principle of best interests may need to be applied rapidly by the doctor and health care team involved and would be considered alongside Article 2 (the right to life) of the Human Rights Act 1998 (see *Section 8.2.3*). As everyone is very different, exactly what a best interests decision should be is not specified in the Mental Capacity Act, which sets out key guiding principles rather than defining what decision should be made. It is important to remember that these are not just medical best interests, and consideration should be given to the person's welfare in a wider sense, thinking about their wishes, values and beliefs in the context of the decision. If this decision is about treatment for a mental health condition, for example depression or psychosis, then it is outside of the scope of the Mental Capacity Act and the Mental Health Act 1983 should be applied (see *Section 8.2.4*).

To support this process a decision-maker needs to be identified, who must be someone who is familiar with the requirements of the Mental Capacity Act. This can be a practitioner or member of the team involved in the delivery of health or social care interventions, the person's own appointed solicitor or a court-appointed deputy. The identification of the most appropriate person to be the decision-maker depends on the nature and severity of the decision and who is most able to make a decision that is in the best interests of the person without bias, considering the wider context of the physical and mental health, beliefs and wishes of the individual. To achieve this, the relationship between the person and decision-maker needs to be collaborative and free from any coercion.

In many situations those most involved in a person's care may be in the best position. However, some points need to be considered: for example, a health care practitioner has an emphasis on preserving life; similarly, a family member may have their own beliefs and wishes, which might lead them to influence the outcome. One option is to request the intervention of an *independent mental capacity advocate*; these are people who have experience and expertise in supporting people with mental illness, dementia, brain injury, etc. with their decision-making, and they are independent of other influences.

The nurse's role is to support this process of decision-making through the sharing of information they know about the person from their records and from contact and communication with the individual and with significant others who know the person well. To do this the Mental Capacity Act lists points you need to consider and enquire about, while at all stages in the process being inclusive of the individual, encouraging and supporting them to participate:

1. Find out the person's current and past views to gain an understanding of their wishes, beliefs and values.
2. Find out from records whether they have previously expressed any wishes at a time when they had capacity. For example, has the person made an advance decision at a point where they had capacity about the treatment or decision proposed?
3. Talk to family members, carers and friends to get to know about the individual.

Before a best interests decision is made to act on behalf of someone who lacks capacity, all factors should be considered, including the perspective and involvement of all the appropriate people. This is often done through a best interests meeting with the person present. The first point considered should always be whether there is a need to make a decision and act on it at all. If a decision does need to be made, then this should be the least restrictive option that achieves the original purpose while allowing the person the most freedom. This is not always possible and where there will be restrictions to the person's freedom the Liberty Protection Safeguards should be put in place.

Liberty Protection Safeguards

These require an application to the local authority, which will review all of the information surrounding the case to ensure that all the steps of the Mental Capacity Act have been followed and the decision is in the person's best interests.

The Liberty Protection Safeguards came into being in response to a 2014 Supreme Court ruling (*P v Cheshire West and Chester Council*) that resulted in an amendment to the Mental Capacity Act Deprivation of Liberty Safeguards (DoLS). They were initially due to pass into UK law on 1 October 2020. However, owing to the challenges faced during the COVID-19 pandemic this was revised to April 2022. The reason for this is to allow for a code of practice to be developed to guide the professionals and organisations responsible for their implementation. It is important to note that the intention of the amendment is not to remove the DoLS, but to make them easier for professionals to interpret and apply, and to include a more robust system for reviewing individual applications. Following the court ruling, a notice was issued advising local authorities of the requirements to take an objective approach and ensure that applications are correctly in place.

The acid test set out by Lady Hale (Law Commission, 2017) provides that the objective element of a deprivation of liberty is satisfied if a person is:
(a) under continuous supervision and control; and
(b) not free to leave.

It is unlawful to decide not to put Liberty Protection Safeguards in place purely because an individual has made no attempt to leave or the person's family is happy with the situation.

These safeguards are more usually applied in an inpatient setting or a care home: for example, a person with dementia may need supervision to keep them safe from harm.

8.2.3 Human Rights Act 1998

Within the legal frameworks, the Human Rights Act 1998 is the UK response in law to the European Convention on Human Rights. It sets out the fundamental rights and principles everyone in the UK is entitled to and can reasonably expect. The key principles to consider in health care are:

- fairness
- respect
- equality
- dignity
- autonomy (choice and control).

These principles are also reflected in the NMC Code (NMC, 2018b) and in the Acts already discussed in this chapter. The Human Rights Act thus influences the standards expected of health and social care services and the professionals working within those services, who must respect the rights of people in their care and treat all individuals with dignity. The rights and freedoms of individuals are included under Part 1 of the Act as articles; those considered most relevant in a health care setting are as follows:

Article 2: Right to life – Anyone who receives health care services has a right to interventions to protect their life. It would be considered unlawful, for example, to withhold a life-saving treatment for an individual or to fail to maintain a person's safety when they did not have the capacity to keep themselves safe, as with the Liberty Protection Safeguards. Article 2 can also apply to neglect that endangers life, for example failing to check that a patient who struggles with eating and drinking is receiving enough fluids and nutrition.

Article 3: Freedom from torture or inhumane and degrading treatment – This links with the Equality Act and considers the principle of dignity. For example, if an individual with dementia was to be made fun of because of their behaviours, this would be considered degrading treatment.

Article 5: Right to liberty and security – This relates also to the Mental Capacity Act: it is unlawful to deprive someone of their ability to leave a health care setting unless there is a clear and valid reason, and the correct safeguards are in place.

Article 8: Right to respect for a private and family life – This is about how we manage information about our patients and respect their confidentiality. It has links to other legislation surrounding data protection.

Article 9: Freedom of thought, conscience and religion – This should be considered with the Equality Act. It is also about respect and ensuring that those who use health care services are included in the planning and decisions about their care. The Human Rights Act also says that people have the right to put their thoughts into action. If the thoughts relate to religion, then they have the right to wear religious clothing and practise their religion. Importantly, patients following some religions and practices (e.g. veganism) refuse certain medications because of the component parts of the medication (e.g. insulin derived from pigs).

Article 14: Prohibition of discrimination – This is linked to the Equality Act and protected characteristics. However, it is also wider, as it encompasses discrimination not included in the protected characteristics that are about differences, for example bullying of an individual because of their appearance and treating everyone with compassion.

These articles help to guide our thinking about the role and responsibilities of nurses, while also starting to consider how ethics and the ethical principles discussed later in this chapter play an important part in supporting actions and decision-making in nursing practice.

8.2.4 Mental Health Act 1983

The Mental Health Act 1983 (as amended in 2007) is legislation developed to give certain health care professionals the powers to detain, assess and treat individuals under specific circumstances, which are defined within the Act.

The Act includes a number of sections to protect individuals and their rights that are applied in mental health care settings and are thus relevant to mental health specialists. They are outside the scope of this book, and in this section we will consider the parts of the Act where adult nurses have a role and need some knowledge and understanding.

In an emergency where it is decided that a person needs immediate care and control, the police have the powers to take that person to a place of safety for an assessment. These powers are:

Section 135 warrant – This is when an individual is in their own home and police need to enter to take the person to a place of safety.

Section 136 warrant – This is when an individual is in a public place and police need to take the person to a safe place.

There are local policies in place to identify the locations of these safe places for the purposes of a mental health assessment. This can sometimes be within an A&E department, and as an adult nurse you may be the first point of contact for the person if they also have needs for physical intervention. The person should not leave until they have been assessed by the mental health team.

There are certain conditions for admission and treatment under the Act. Under the civil procedures, to be admitted for assessment under the amended Act (section 2) a person must be:
(a) suffering from a mental disorder of a nature or degree which warrants the detention of the patient in hospital for assessment (or for assessment followed by medical treatment) for at least a limited period; and
(b) the person ought to be so detained in the interests of their own health or safety or with a view to the protection of other persons.

To be admitted for treatment under the amended Act (section 3):

(a) a person must be suffering from a mental disorder of a nature or degree which makes it appropriate for him to receive medical treatment in a hospital; and

(b) it is necessary for the health and safety of the patient or for the protection of other persons that he should receive such treatment and it cannot be provided unless he is detained under this section; and

(c) appropriate medical treatment is available for the person.

The decision concerning the application of the Mental Health Act must be made by three appropriate professionals with the knowledge and skills to make a decision. These are an *approved mental health professional* (AMHP) (this may be a mental health nurse or a social worker who has completed additional training), a *doctor* who knows the person (usually their GP) and an *approved doctor* (usually a psychiatrist). There are usually mental health liaison teams working with A&E departments to support the assessment of individuals where there are concerns that they need treatment for their mental health – if treatment is needed, the individual would be admitted to a mental health inpatient setting. The involvement for adult nursing is in the referral for assessment and ensuring that physical health care needs are met in the A&E department or if they initially require admission to an acute medical ward, for example following an overdose.

8.3 Ethics

A wise person once said, 'If you want an easy life... do *not* study ethics'. Ethics comes from the Greek word 'ethos', which means habit, character or disposition. In philosophical terms, Beauchamp and Childress (2019) describe ethics as being about the way we think, understand and decide how best to lead a moral life. The concept of ethics has been influenced over the ages by religions and different cultures, debated by well-known philosophers such as Plato, Aristotle, Kant and Mill, and although we can use ethics to justify the decisions we make, the outcome of the use of ethics in practice may not be that transparent or palatable to all.

Ethics set out our moral code or the principles that individuals and societies follow. Ethics influence how we live our lives and the way in which we care for our clients. Ethical debates on topics such as animal rights, euthanasia, war and abortion can be explored using ethical theories and principles. Moral uncertainty or ambiguity is difficult: as humans we would prefer there to be one right answer, and as professionals we are required to take responsibility for the decisions we make and behaviours we show. Developing an understanding of the ethical issues will therefore help you pinpoint aspects of the moral problems people argue about.

Ethical theories and principles can help us view things from a different perspective, removing emotion from the debate. Understanding ethical frameworks may help us find some common ground in which agreement can be reached or may direct us towards a possible solution to a problem.

You need to keep in mind that ethics will not give one single right answer, but an ethical framework can help to clarify issues and eliminate some confusion.

It might even lead to several right answers or fewer wrong ones. It can help us make and justify a decision, but it does not absolve us of the responsibility of making a decision. Essentially, an ethical framework enables us in most ways to distinguish right from wrong, but this is also influenced by our own moral judgement. Such a judgement may be sited in a health care frame, where health, illness, care and treatment are often at odds in a single case. Although you can try to remove emotion from the decisions you make, even when you are making the 'right' ethical/moral decision, it will not always make you feel comfortable with the outcome.

ACTIVITY 8.1

Consider two patient scenarios involving end of life care. One patient is given treatment; the other is not. One patient lacked capacity; the other did not. What factors do you feel may have been considered in arriving at the decisions made? Are you comfortable with them?

8.4 **Ethical theories**

Ethical theory is constructed on a golden rule that guides us as to how we should live, namely:

'We should do to others what we want others to do to us.'

If we take this at its most basic level, I want people to be nice and friendly to me, therefore I will be nice and friendly to them. That sounds simple, yet philosophers do not all agree and there are therefore many hybrid positions or theories around this golden rule. Three common strands to these hybrid positions are known as the ethical theories of *deontology* and *consequentialism*, both of which try to guide us as to what we morally should do or be forbidden from doing, and *virtue ethics*, which asks us to focus on a person's character and development and which some virtue theorists believe can guide us as to how we should behave.

8.4.1 **Deontological theory**

This is a duty-based theory in which we will follow our obligations to others or society, as this is the ethically correct thing to do. For example, if I make a promise then I will keep that promise. I will not break the law, and the decisions I make will be consistent, no matter the circumstances. I will have acted from a sense of duty, and the motive for my action is judged more important than the action or consequence. Therefore, an intervention for the right reason, even if the outcome is terrible, would be viewed as the right thing to do.

A flaw in the theory is that we can never fully know the intent of the person making the decision and thus cannot define whether they acted morally or not. For example, if I hand over a stolen bike, is it because I have a duty to society (morally right) or is it really for the reward money (morally wrong)?

When we consider duty, we have no clear basis to define when a duty starts and ends, nor what happens if two duties conflict with each other. For example, if a nurse is driving to visit a patient and is late for the visit, they have a duty both to the patient to be on time and to society to follow the rules of the road and not to speed. Which duty has the higher priority?

Deontology is often associated with the German philosopher Immanuel Kant (1724–1804). Kantian ethics proposed that as rational human beings we have certain duties: we should treat other people always as an end and never a means to an end. In other words, we should not use other people for our own gain and we should always recognise their humanity. Kant argued that we act morally from a sense of duty. This duty should not be influenced by past experiences of an individual or our own personal bias. Such an application of duty may lead to consistent and understandable care where all are treated similarly.

8.4.2 Consequentialism and utilitarianism

Consequentialism is a goal-based theory that suggests that an action is morally right if the consequence of that action is more favourable than unfavourable. Unlike deontology, the result of the action is the sole determining factor and can be easily measured. This makes it a quick way to morally assess an action, as it is based on experience as opposed to intuition or duty. The outcome can be measured or seen to be morally right, whereas people's motives cannot.

Within consequentialism we have some subdivisions:
- **Egoism** – the action is morally right if the consequences of that action are more favourable to the person performing the act (as before, returning the stolen bike is right and I get a reward).
- **Altruism** – the action is morally right if the consequence of that action is more favourable to everyone except the person performing the act (e.g. giving £10 to feed homeless people: as I'm not homeless I will not get fed and I'm £10 poorer).
- **Utilitarianism** – the action is morally right if the consequences are more favourable to the greatest number of people.

Utilitarianism differs slightly from consequentialism in that utilitarianism requires a specific desired outcome. Jeremy Bentham (1748–1832) and John Stuart Mill (1806–1873) are known as the founders of utilitarianism. Bentham created his own definition of human nature, called the happiness sum: 'it is the greatest happiness of the greatest number that is the measure of right and wrong'. He believed that humans would seek pleasure and avoid pain.

Mill was a student of Bentham, but he did not agree with everything his teacher taught him. He viewed utilitarianism as a theory promoting the argument that actions are right in proportion.

Mill is sometimes described as a 'rule utilitarian', as he accepted that we have a sense of duty to stick to traditional moral rules, but that flexibility is required. Therefore, some behaviours are morally wrong if they do not produce the greatest happiness for the greatest number of people. Mill stated that a healthy society would be made up of a huge variety of different individuals and lifestyles, with room for those who are outside the norm. If they do not interfere with the freedoms of others, people should be allowed to think and do what they like.

A flaw in this theory is that if most of the population feel that people with mental illness should be detained in hospitals then that becomes the greatest happiness for the greatest number of people – and that is what will happen.

8.4.3 Virtue ethics

Virtue ethics is one of the oldest normative traditional theories used in Western philosophy. It requires a person to be judged by their character rather than their actions. This ethical theory has been in decline as our understanding of human behaviour has developed. As an example, a psychopath who has harmed others but has the character to be charming and hard working in society would be viewed as a good person based on their character; their action of hurting others clearly contradicts this view.

Virtue ethics is focused on developing good habits and morals in childhood, as taught by parents and adults. Plato identified the cardinal virtues of wisdom, courage, temperance and justice, and advocated avoiding vices such as cowardice, injustice and vanity. What we need to consider when discussing virtues and vices is what the right amount is. For example, if I develop too much courage, I may become egocentric and rash; not enough and I might be classed as a coward.

If we consider moral development, a flaw in this theory is that sometimes good parents have children who do wrong. In addition, once we develop good morals, will we always behave in a moral way? Or do our thoughts, feelings and experiences influence our behaviour at times in such a way that may cause us to be immoral? By following this theory as prescribed, if I pass a homeless person in the street and give them a pound, it would then be immoral of me to not give a pound to every homeless person I pass.

Despite the theory's flaws and its decline, virtue ethics still has resonance in health care. As nurses, we help care for and treat people who may think, feel and behave in a manner outside the norm or not acceptable in society. They may behave that way for a variety of reasons, some of which have developed in childhood. The learning from virtue ethics allows us to develop a non-judgemental approach, treating people as equals. It helps us to focus on the person's character and not their behaviour or actions related to their mental illness.

ACTIVITY 8.2

If we think about the NHS, many people say it runs on a utilitarian basis. Why do you think this is and what would be the difficulty if it ran on the basis of the other ethical theories?

8.4.4 Biomedical ethics

Beauchamp and Childress (2019) developed a framework made up of four moral principles that can guide practitioners in managing aspects of their practice that cause confusion and conflict:

- autonomy

- beneficence
- non-maleficence
- justice.

Despite some debate, they are cross-cultural (Ebbesen, Andersen and Pedersen, 2012) and still used today to guide patients and professionals in ethical dilemmas within health care. The principles must be fulfilled in every situation if they do not conflict with each other, which is referred to as *'prima facie* binding'.

If they do conflict, then this raises a moral obligation that no simple set of moral principles can easily address. Beauchamp and Childress (2019) highlight the case of a psychiatrist needing to balance his knowledge that the appointment of a person in whose confidence he is might cause problems for the new employer but be beneficial for the person. It is anticipated that the four moral principles may help to clarify the thoughts behind the decision. But, can they create a hard and fast set of rules for what he must or should do?

We will look at each principle in turn.

Autonomy

The people in our care have a right to choose the care and treatment they receive. Recognition of this has seen the NHS make huge strides over the past few years to ensure that people have more of a say not only in the care and treatment they receive but also with regard to where they wish to receive it (NHS, 2021). An aim of autonomy is to give people maximum liberty in devising their own lives and values (Callahan, 2003). None of us are perfect in the decisions we make, but that does not take away the right we have to make these decisions, as Principle 3 of the Mental Capacity Act 2005 makes clear with regard to unwise decisions.

Informed consent and confidentiality are just two examples in which health care professionals respect people's autonomy. We make a promise that we will only do to patients what they have agreed to, and that the information patients share with us will be private and the limits to that privacy would only be breached if they have harmed themselves or others or there is the risk that they will do so. Therefore, a key to respecting autonomy is good communication and active listening skills so we are clear as to our patients' wishes.

One philosophy, inherent in solution-focused therapy and commonly applied in much of the mental health field, is to ensure that we respect autonomy and that people are always treated as 'experts in their own life' (De Jong and Berg, 2002). In other words people have the knowledge and skills to help themselves: for example, when we get angry, the strategies we use to calm ourselves are not always the same strategies that work for others.

'Paternalism' describes a doctor–patient or nurse–patient relationship in which the doctor or nurse acts as if they know what is best for the patient (Lepping, Palmstierna and Raveesh, 2016). It can result in interventions and practice without consultation or against the patient's wishes even if the patient does not lack the capacity to give consent. Effective communication and listening while respecting autonomy will aid individualised care and treatment and a move away from paternalism.

For individuals who lack decision-making capacity we must work on a 'decision-by-decision' basis and never on the assumption that the person lacks capacity for every decision. We need to consider how we uphold their autonomy, ensuring that we obtain the patient's view where possible and that any intervention undertaken is in their best interests, which supports the principles of beneficence and non-maleficence.

Beneficence

A definition of beneficence is 'always doing good'. In health care this can mean that we should always seek to do the best for the people in our care, and as health care professionals it is a given that we enter into this profession to care and do good for others in need. Yet we still have incidents of harm caused to patients in the health care system. This may be a result of paternalism, but in mental health care often our patients have lost contact with reality and in doing good we may cause harm. In that case we must consider the principle of non-maleficence.

Non-maleficence

Non-maleficence means 'doing no harm'. Beauchamp and Childress (2019) link this to the nature of health care by arguing that we 'ought' to do things that cause no harm. You may also hear the Latin phrase *primum non nocere* ('first do no harm').

An example of this is when care or treatment are given against the person's wishes as they are deemed to be in the person's best interests and supported by legislation, such as holding someone down to give treatment, or preventing someone's liberty for the safety of themselves and others. It is logical to say that beneficence and non-maleficence are intertwined and we might assume that if we are doing good by someone then we are not harming them. Yet the drugs we give may have severe side effects, injections puncture the skin and cause physical harm, and the restrictions we place on the person can cause psychological harm. Although legislation protects and supports us in doing the least harm for potential good, we must never lose sight of the patient's experience and the possibility that the treatment may feel unjust in some way.

Justice

In health care we associate justice with fairness. Gillon (2003) subdivided the obligation of justice into three parts:
- morally acceptable laws (legal justice)
- respect for people's rights arising from the legislation discussed in *Section 8.2* (rights-based justice)
- fair distribution of scarce resources (distributive justice).

We are all aware that the NHS does not have an infinite amount of money. It must provide care and treatment to the public within stringent budgets, ensuring as far as possible equal access to the same level of health care regardless of where someone lives. Equality is at the very centre of the principle of justice and, although the Equality Act 2010 clarifies these issues, health care professionals not only to balance the needs of each patient in their care, but also to decide on which patients take priority, while trying to provide equal access, keep within their budget and still allow for patient choice (autonomy).

Sometimes these principles are in conflict. As there are finite resources available, somebody somewhere may not get their life-saving treatment because ten other people require a different life-saving treatment. Doing good (beneficence) by ten people outweighs the harm done to one, as it is the least harmful course of action (non-maleficence). However, it is unjust for the person who misses out, as both treatments should be available (justice). Respect for people's autonomy requires us to know the views of the one patient, as they may choose to die to let the others live. We see here the principles of both utilitarianism – in the greatest good for the greatest number – and deontology – if the person has the maxim of dying so that others can live, then the decision would be morally correct.

Health care professionals are often required to make difficult decisions, some of which challenge us ethically and have both an emotional and professional impact on us. Understanding the legal and ethical frameworks in which we work can help us to make those decisions.

ACTIVITY 8.3

Once you have developed your understanding on each of the moral principles, attempt to specify, determine and balance some often contentious issues in health care practice, e.g. euthanasia, abortion.

CHAPTER SUMMARY

Key points to take away from *Chapter 8*:
- ☑ There are many different legal frameworks to consider.
- ☑ Health care in the UK is based on human rights principles that are in turn reflected in European legislation.
- ☑ Acts of Parliament (statutes) provide mandatory rules and regulations related to specific situations.
- ☑ Ethical health care practice is largely founded on four principles: autonomy, beneficence, non-maleficence and justice.

Questions

Question 8.1	What is the golden rule of ethics in health care? *(Learning outcome 8.2)*
Question 8.2	How can a nurse's actions aid the decision-making process in any capacity assessment and implementation? *(Learning outcome 8.1)*
Question 8.3	What are the specific characteristics of the Equality Act? *(Learning outcome 8.1)*
Question 8.4	What would the outcome be if nurses failed to follow Acts (statutes)? *(Learning outcome 8.3)*
Question 8.5	Describe themes related to moral duty in nursing. *(Learning outcomes 8.1, 8.2, 8.3)*

FURTHER READING

Cuthbert, S. and Quallington, J. (2017) *Values and Ethics for Care Practice*. Lantern Publishing.

Department for Constitutional Affairs (2013) *Mental Capacity Act Code of Practice*. Available at: www.gov.uk/government/publications/mental-capacity-act-code-of-practice (accessed 23 June 2021).

NHS (2021) *Mental Capacity Act*. Available at: www.nhs.uk/conditions/social-care-and-support-guide/making-decisions-for-someone-else/mental-capacity-act (accessed 23 June 2021).

NHS (2021) *Involving People in Their Own Care*. Available at: www.england.nhs.uk/ourwork/patient-participation (accessed 23 June 2021).

Schultz, P.L. and Baker, J. (2017) Teaching strategies to increase nursing student acceptance and management of unconscious bias. *Journal of Nursing Education*, **56(11)**: 692–6.

UK Government (2021) *Understanding Legislation*. Available at: www.legislation.gov.uk/understanding-legislation (accessed 23 June 2021).

Veesart, A. and Barron, A. (2020) Unconscious bias: is it impacting your nursing care? *Nursing Made Incredibly Easy!* **18(2)**: 47–9.

Chapter 9
Risk

Neil Murphy

LEARNING OUTCOMES

By the end of this chapter you should be able to:

9.1 Understand the concept of risk

9.2 Describe the process and elements of assessing risk

9.3 Articulate factors influencing the presence (static and dynamic) of risk in patients

9.4 List factors related to risk of violence and suicide

9.5 Reflect on how risk affects an individual and develop a simple formulation (explanation) for their risk.

9.1 Introduction

Risk is a concept that has many meanings that can relate to various situations, and in this chapter the focus is in relation to health. Generally, definitions of risk contain reference to potential danger, loss or injury. But the potential of risk (e.g. history of self-harm or violence that is not evident at the time) does not always need to relate to a physical event: risk can relate to values, rights and opportunities.

Risk is linked to a variety of things in our lives and often we are unaware of its presence. The hidden influence of risk can affect how much insurance you pay for your home or car. Risk is involved in your employment and in your recruitment to any future role. It is also identifiable in the lifestyle you adopt and in many of the decisions you take.

- Risk can be a planned event – for example, a young person may be offered car insurance on a high-powered car but it will come at some financial cost.
- It can be unplanned – for example, employing people to take on a role and finding that they are unable to fulfil the role, leading to plans not being achieved.
- It can be predictable – for example, if you have an ageing employment base and you do not plan for people leaving through retirement (and still need the same number of staff) then you will be short of staff.

- Finally, it can be unpredictable and uncontrollable – for example, arriving at work to find that the rest of the team have all independently left a message that they cannot come in today, so an order due to be completed cannot be fulfilled.

All the above factors will probably resonate with your experiences. The perception of risk involves each individual and their subjective view of something negative happening because of some factor they have encountered. It is intuitive in many cases, but the skill to assess and manage risk can be developed from this initial intuition. Often you will have a sense of unease and foreboding. Such senses are commonly related to you perceiving something that you are uncomfortable with or find confusing and potentially threatening to you. Each person will view an event in a unique and individual way. The way you view something is governed by many factors, but primarily by experience and knowledge. Therefore, if you think something is going to be risky, you will react in the way that you have learnt to react to risky events.

Risk can be interpreted in a negative and frightening way, but it can also be interpreted as excitement. The key theme here is that there is some interpretation that is related to you as an individual. The way you react to the risk may lead to learned actions for the future, in a way of coping. For example, if you are late for work, you might drive at an uncomfortable speed but arrive in work in sufficient time not to be noticed by your manager. The cognitive reaction to the risk of driving uncomfortably fast leads you to feel that you can take such a risk again, each time becoming accustomed to the feelings until they are not uncomfortable but potentially enjoyable.

A major problem that health care workers encounter is that they cannot avoid risk. In most forms of health care, risk needs to be assessed (e.g. triage carried out in an A&E department, a patient refusing to take their medication). The way you feel about and interpret risk and your level of experience will influence the way you assess and deal with the risk.

In mental health care, risk assessment is often related to having to remove decision-making from a risky individual. This may involve giving fewer options, so as to provide a clear direction to address any risk, or in some circumstances detaining people against their wishes. The removal of decision-making may indirectly give more ownership of a risk back to the person, by enabling them (if possible) to see that there was an alternative way to addressing the risk that may have been different from their initial choice but resulted in no harm. The next section will explore risk and risk assessment in mental health care as related to direct personal care.

9.2 Assessing risk

Risk is defined, in relation to health, as the likelihood, imminence and severity of a negative event occurring: for example, violence, self-harm or self-neglect (Department of Health, 2009). The art of assessing risk has been explored over many years by many authors, but specifically by Monahan and Steadman, and the MacArthur Foundation, culminating in them suggesting that risk assessment is usually seen as attempts to predict risk (e.g. see Monahan *et al.*, 2001). The many and varied areas related to risk are frequently researched, and UK national statistics are produced annually – for example, the National Confidential Inquiry into Suicide and Safety in Mental Health (NCISH) project, based at the University of Manchester, has collected information about all suicides in the UK since 1996. Despite this, many clinicians remain a little unsure about the best way to assess risk. Much of the evidence for this is seen in the research debates related to the value of assessing risk (see Szmukler and Rose, 2013) and the many and varied tools created to assess risk (see University of Manchester, 2018).

Guidance from the Royal College of Psychiatrists (RCPsych, 2016) suggests that risk assessment must acknowledge its dynamic nature and that risk is subject to changes in presentation over short periods of time. Just as risk can change over time, so historically has the approach to assessing risk. Risk assessment and management in mental health care is commonly influenced by adverse events, such as the death of Rocky Bennett, who suffocated while being restrained in the prone position, a 'traditional' restraint at the time (Mind, 2013, p. 3).

Much current practice related to risk assessment and management is found in the Department of Health's *Best Practice in Managing Risk* (Department of Health, 2009). Its guidance in many areas is used throughout this chapter and many NHS Trust policies are linked to this best practice advice.

There are some key concepts in assessing risk:
- Risk is a normal thing to encounter in our everyday life.
- Risk can be 'static' or 'dynamic' (each will be developed later in the chapter).
- The Department of Health (2009) argues that risk assessment is a sensitive topic and one that can be challenging; I would further argue that this is the case for both the person being assessed and the people assessing.
- The NMC (2018b) argues that nurses should, where possible, aim to protect people who may be at risk or are considered vulnerable from harm, neglect or abuse.

ACTIVITY 9.1

What risks do you think you face in your everyday life? Think about the past few days and write them down.

9.2.1 Static risk

Static risks are usually unchanging and often referred to as historic risk – for example, a history of childhood neglect or a history of self-harm.

Mental health risk assessment has focused on historical factors that have been seen repeatedly in groups of people (e.g. in age groups, professions, in relation to past risk behaviours). Service response has been aimed at reducing risks as a way of protecting people. One way of achieving this is to remove responsibility for their actions from the person at risk. However, by taking responsibility for maintaining safety instead of enabling the person at risk to develop the skills to do so for themselves, services can in some cases increase the risk rather than diminish it.

ACTIVITY 9.2

How do you think that mental health services may act with a person who said that they were at risk of suicide? Write down your thoughts.

9.2.2 Dynamic risk

Dynamic risk is fluid and can include a person's mental state and lifestyle choices. Dynamic risks are ever-changing.

It is normal for people to feel that life is not good at times, and some people who have limited cognitive ability or life experience articulate these thoughts as feeling suicidal. Someone feeling as though they may be suicidal does not always equate to someone who is actively suicidal and at a high level of risk. Just because someone states that they feel suicidal does not mean that they are actively wanting to end their life. However, a nurse needs to accept that the person may be suicidal, establish in what way they are at risk and report this information immediately to a senior colleague, ensuring that the person remains safe.

The NMC argues that, as a nurse, you need to accept that people who may be, or state that they may be, at risk have the right to refuse or not take part in treatment, but that you will need to act in their best interests (see *Section 8.2.1*). That may not be a simple linear action. Often the nurse needs to involve other professionals, but such a decision may require them to share confidential information with others who the person may not want the nurse to speak to (see *Section 9.4* on safeguarding). This decision does not fall to the student nurse, but information gathered by a student nurse may be important to more senior staff's decision to share confidential information with other professionals.

9.2.3 Factors influencing the risk of suicide and violence

Although there are many other factors related to risk in mental health presentations, violence and suicide are discussed next. The reason for this is that both are reported in national statistics each year. *Table 9.1* highlights some of the key areas of information gathered over many years that have been found to contribute to the risk of violence and suicide. The table shows only a modified short version of the information available and is used for indicative purposes (more comprehensive data is collected by the NCISH; see also Department of Health, 2009).

Table 9.1 *Factors influencing the risk of violence and suicide*

	Violence	**Suicide**
Demographics	Young age Male Employment problems	Increasing age Male Unemployment Living alone
History	History of violence Childhood maltreatment	History of self-harm (also family history of suicide) History of abuse History of mental illness
Clinical history	Psychopathy/personality disorder Non-adherence to treatment	Diagnosis of mental illness (e.g. depression, personality disorder, schizophrenia) Contact (may have been recently discharged) with psychiatric services Physical illness
Psychological	Impulsivity Anger and suspicion Violent attitude Lack of insight into problem	Impulsivity Hopelessness and lack of self-esteem Lack of support Life event
Current context	Threatening Access to weapons	Suicidal and has plans Access to means Lethality of means

9.2.4 Risk of vulnerability

Amendments to the Mental Health Act in 2007 suggest that people leaving a mental health hospital should continue to receive help because of their potential vulnerability. Vulnerability related to mental illness is seen in people who may be exploitable and are at risk of being victimised. This is associated with people being intimidated, bullied and, in some instances, abused. Care is needed to consider such vulnerability, to assess each person for the potential for such risk and to explore ways to manage any identified risks. Importantly, empowering the individual to have a voice and articulate how things are for them is inherent in developing an accurate assessment. A person might be victimised by others simply because they have a mental health problem or even because they are on medication.

9.2.5 Risk of self-neglect

Many of the tools designed for assessing risk in the mentally unwell include sections that focus on neglect (by the self and others) (see Morgan, 2000).

Self-neglect can take many forms, but is often associated with some form of deficient behaviour, such as lack of self-care or unconscious omission of action that might impinge on the person's health. Care is needed not to confuse a risk behaviour that has some conscious action (e.g. deliberately not taking medication) and someone's unconscious omission or action due to confusion or preoccupation.

> **ACTIVITY 9.3**
>
> In what ways do you believe that having a mental illness may cause vulnerability or self-neglect? Write down your thoughts.

9.3 Considerations in assessing risk

To make further sense of the risks detailed in this chapter it was found simplest to use the headings from *Best Practice in Managing Risk* (Department of Health, 2009) to frame the discussion in this section.

9.3.1 History

As can be seen from many of the risk assessment tools, such as the 20-item Historical–Clinical–Risk Management scale, version 3 (HCR-20V3) (Douglas *et al.*, 2013), and from static risk factors, a history of a person presenting with risks is a major predictor in the person posing a risk again. Many of the risks people present with are related to their past behaviour, such as substance misuse, alcohol use, self-neglect, use of violence or self-harm. Knowledge of these historical behaviours can be beneficial for the nurse and the patient, but it may also cause a problem for both.

> **ACTIVITY 9.4**
>
> What potential problems could happen if a health care worker has knowledge of a person's past risk-related behaviour? Write down your thoughts.

A history of violence or self-harm are often seen as powerful predictors of a person's potential to be violent or to self-harm in the future. However, just because a person has a history of risky behaviour, this should not mean that they should be constantly viewed as posing a risk. Care is needed to establish the risks present and to see whether a pattern of risk from the past is happening again. Often on further investigation a trigger to such behaviours can be found and this can be seen as an early warning sign for the potential risk.

Key themes that should be considered are:

- a relationship between becoming mentally unwell and the use of violence or self-harm
- a lack of tolerance and a level of impulsivity
- an increase in stress for the person, which could be social, familial or environmental.

There are several things that should be looked for when assessing historical risks:

- What has stopped the risks from being actualised?
- What has changed between the period of being 'well' and now 'becoming unwell'?
- Are the risks following a pattern seen before?

9.3.2 Environment

If a person has been living in an environment where certain behaviours are acceptable (as a member of a gang, for example), then some of their displayed actions and coping strategies may not conform to the expectations of others outside of that environment. Similarly, if someone has been in a hospital environment, has a military background, has been in prison or has had some long-term exile from societal influences, then their behaviour and their understanding of society may be compromised. A person from such environments may present with risky behaviours, but may also be at risk because they do not understand currently acceptable societal behaviours.

It is important to remember as well that hospital environments do have specific levels of risk attached to them. People in such environments may be vulnerable and others can exploit and take advantage of them both in hospital and on returning to their usual place of living. For some, remaining in hospital may seem a safe solution to either the risks they pose or the risks they are vulnerable to. But the longer a person remains in a hospital environment, the longer their skills for life may become compromised and coping strategies altered and modified to fit with that environment.

9.3.3 Mental state

The symptoms of some mental disorders can increase the risks the person poses both to themselves and to others. Symptoms related to the belief that someone controls them or is intending to harm them or that they have unique abilities that they do not have (delusional beliefs) can cause some people to act or place themselves in precarious situations where harm may occur. Alongside this, the strength of their belief may cause an increase in anger or suspiciousness if others contradict their viewpoint. Commonly, behaviours become less predictable, and the person can lose any insight and capacity to control their responses. Here an increase in symptoms can be seen to increase risks, with the person becoming more unwell and often less engaged with care providers or carers.

Occasionally, a person's mental state can become so entrenched in misperceptions that they stop caring for themselves and actively avoid contact. Reinforcement by the actions of others can lead to further entrenchment and a spiralling downwards of mental health.

9.3.4 Information from others

Carers and friends can illuminate changes that have occurred recently in a person who is becoming unwell. Often, such people have essential knowledge of the person's usual practice and behaviour and their coping strategies and, more importantly, awareness of deterioration in health. Care is needed not to ignore any information related to risk. An important factor for the nurse is not to appear to be favouring service perspectives over those of clients or carers, as this may inadvertently antagonise the situation. Carers are important people in the recovery of someone who has a mental health difficulty. These people are in frequent contact with the individual and provide support by offering more time and encouragement than a health care professional can ever offer.

9.3.5 Clinical judgement

A relatively recent addition to risk assessment is the inclusion of clinical judgement. Clinical judgement has a range of factors that need to be considered. Nurses need to have knowledge of all fields of health presentation, and your undergraduate training is intended to equip you with the fundamentals. However, when you are qualified and working in adult physical care, knowledge about mental health may become a little faded. The judgement an adult nurse needs to demonstrate includes the ability to reflect on personal experience of working with people with a mental health problem, taking into account other patients they may have met in the past who presented in a similar way. The nurse also needs to establish what risks the nurse, the patient and the carer may feel are present and decide, once sufficient information has been gathered, who to discuss the risk with further.

An important factor regarding clinical judgement is that it is only one component of the way that the nurse will establish the level of risks. Acting only on clinical judgement without historic information and standard risk information will mean that any risk assessment is limited in its value. However, the combination has been seen to complement the accuracy of assessments and is seen in more recent risk assessment tools (Douglas *et al.*, 2013). The health care professional's knowledge and understanding can, when paired with a structured tool, have more accuracy and be more meaningful to all in its outcomes. The process also enables confirmation by the patient and their involvement in establishing a formulation (understanding or explanation) of how things link together in their unique life.

9.4 Safeguarding

Safeguarding is an essential area for discussion in any health or social care service. Much of the focus is on the protection of the person's wellbeing and their human rights. So far in this chapter, safeguarding issues have been identified without direct reference to, but hopefully with an implication of, partnership in establishing the risks. The sections related to vulnerability (*Section 9.2.4*) and neglect (*Section 9.2.5*) have raised themes related to potential exploitation and quality of life. In this section the focus is realigned to themes involved in any safeguarding discussion: abuse and, in more detail, neglect.

A brief overview of exemplars of both abuse and neglect is offered in the rest of this section (see *Activity 9.6*) to aid identification of key areas and to supplement understanding with regard to risk. *Figure 9.1* shows the main themes.

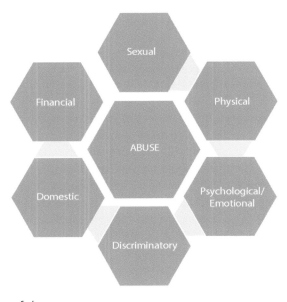

Figure 9.1 *Key areas of abuse.*

ACTIVITY 9.5

List some potential safeguarding issues related to the themes in *Figure 9.1*. Write down your thoughts.

Although each area is identified separately, in some cases one area is implicit in another. For example, domestic abuse may have psychological/emotional factors involved, financial abuse can involve domestic and psychological/emotional abuse.

Neglect is a simple term that has many complicated connotations. Neglect can be under the control of an individual, a deliberate act, and can also relate to personal values and raise cultural and professional challenges.

ACTIVITY 9.6

Can you identify whether the following are examples of neglect?

- Ben is a 16-year-old person who has a heart condition and depression and who will not take his medication. His parents have been found to be grinding some medication and adding it to his food.
- Sally is a 60-year-old person who has been removed from a GP's list for over-attendance. She has a long-term health problem and cannot understand why her behaviour is a problem or why she cannot see the GP when she wants to.
- Sna is a 20-year-old person who has taken a large overdose and has deteriorating neurological signs of life, but breathes independently. Doctors identify a chest infection but decide not to treat it.
- Billy is a 40-year-old person who has stopped putting his garbage out for collection; instead, he hoards it in his house. He stores the refuse in sealed plastic bags in his home and his neighbours continually leave rude messages on his door.

Throughout this section (including *Activity 9.6*), there are many answers, and the nurse will start to consider how to make sense of each one. To manage such instances the Department of Health (2011b) advocates a stepped approach in which the first necessity is to identify safeguarding events. Once identified, there would need to be an assessment to establish the issues and people involved, then the development of some response. Ultimately the local authority in the area where the event takes place will have a specific protocol to enact such safeguarding (e.g. see Local Government Association, 2018). As a health care professional, you will need to be aware of such protocols and may need to raise concerns. Hart's (2014) pocket guide to risk assessment and management for practitioners is a simple reference guide that supplements this chapter.

9.5 **Boundaries**

Within the concept of risk, boundaries of individuals, services and others are important. After all, levels of confidentiality and professionalism are expected from professionals, but what boundaries exist in the eyes of the person receiving care? With respect to risk assessment, they have the right to know of any decisions made for them and to be involved in any risk assessment and development of a management plan.

Care is needed with risk, as some people's behaviour and risk factors can involve others. The nurse needs to explore such instances but also to be vigilant not to breach confidentiality inadvertently when sharing information on identified risks. It is a natural feeling to consider sharing risk details with people who may be involved in the care of the person (such as a relative) or have some vested interest (e.g. a police officer), but the first step would be to discuss and share with senior staff involved in the person's care in order to establish the best route forward.

Also, importantly, sharing risk information with others who are not involved in the care or management of care could breach the rights of the person concerned and not adhere to the General Data Protection Regulation (GDPR) (for guidance see Information Commissioner's Office, 2018).

9.6 **Mass media**

Mass media have played a part in educating and informing people about the risks associated with mental illness. Although selective in nature, the media commonly offer some sound and clear messages related to public health issues and the impact of mental ill health on performance. Campaigns such as Time to Change, led by Mind and Rethink Mental Illness, have been in existence for many years, yet many people are only recently becoming aware of them and their focus on mental health. The reasons for this probably include increased media publicising of World Mental Health Day (10th October) and celebrity acknowledgement and public sharing of experiences of mental ill health.

It is important to highlight some of the issues perhaps missed by the lack of publicising of Time to Change, where it was argued that the mentally ill are more at risk from people without mental illness and from themselves than the general public is at risk from the mentally ill. Although the general public increasingly associates violence with mental ill health, in fact the rate of violence in the mentally unwell has remained constant since the 1990s. In all forms of violence, the most common denominators are drugs and alcohol, not mental ill health. The Time to Change campaign is no longer running, but it continues to maintain a government-funded website offering advice related to mental ill health – see www.time-to-change.org.uk.

Unfortunately, much of the media's representation of mental ill health is still negative. Negative representation is seen in particular in relation to people with schizophrenia and implied drug misuse (Murphy, Fatoye and Wibberley, 2013). Such negative representations have been found to influence practitioners' opinions and actions in a restrictive fashion (Murphy, 2015), causing them to look for risks even when none are indicated.

Public attitudes have been influenced by media reporting over many years. An example is seen in a study by Appleby and Wessely (1988). This happened to be in progress at the time of the Hungerford massacre, a series of random shootings by Michael Ryan (a man initially labelled mentally ill) in August 1987. Before the incident, they had been asking people their opinions about the mentally ill and found that most cared about and wanted a more inclusive approach to help people with a mental health problem to reintegrate into society. The research continued after the incident, with opinion changing to wanting the mentally ill to be separated for public safety. Around six months later the research found that opinion had reverted to the original findings for care and inclusion.

This theme of acceptance and then rejection may be stimulated by media reporting, but it may also be influenced by repressed thoughts and stigmatised views related to trust. This is seen in many examples where the public have resisted the placing of mental health units in their local area, citing fears of danger and risk from the mentally ill. Yet public consultations and representations by service user forums have become the method of addressing fears and have enabled many new community mental health units to be built and become part of the fabric of future mental health care (e.g. see Sussex Partnership NHS Foundation Trust, 2019).

9.7 Practicalities of the assessment of risk

The Department of Health (2009) argues that risk assessment needs to be based in a sensitive way on individual presentation and to take into account individual need and ability. No assessment of risk can be accurately completed without the person who presents with the risk, or without having assessed a range of other factors: the person's social context, their clinical history (both past and current mental health problems) and their own understanding of factors influencing the way they feel at the moment.

9.7.1 Process of developing an understanding and management of risk

The Department of Health (2009) directs health care professionals to use a five-step cyclical model for assessing risk (*Figure 9.2*).

The cycle aims to involve the person who presents with the risk in all decisions at all stages. The process begins with an assessment of the individual emerging risk, how it is seen by the person and others and how it can escalate. Then an agreed plan to manage the risk is put in place, monitored and reviewed for effectiveness. The cycle is then repeated for existing or new risks.

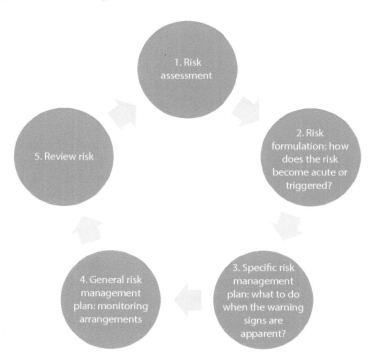

Figure 9.2 *A five-step model for assessing risk and planning risk management (Department of Health, 2009). Reproduced under an Open Government Licence 3.0.*

9.7.2 Application of risk assessment and management to a person

Over the chapters in this book, you will have looked at a range of aspects influencing how mental illness is both presented and viewed. The final section of this chapter provides you with an opportunity to link some of these themes, ranging from a specific type of presentation to an understanding of risk to an individual person.

Scenario: Stephen

Stephen is an 18-year-old person who has presented at A&E with chest pain. He has been to the department many times over the past month. He appears poorly nourished and in a dishevelled state.

ACTIVITY 9.7

What is the first thing you think the nurse engages in with Stephen? Write down your thoughts.

In assessing Stephen, the triage nurse establishes that he has been to the department before for similar difficulties, but also asks whether there was any medical history in his past and any family history of mental illness. Stephen says that he had been in hospital as a child and was supported by the CAMHS team. He says that his brother took his own life when Stephen was 14 years old, also that his mother has had CBT over the past two years after coming off antidepressant drugs.

ACTIVITY 9.8

What are CAMHS teams? What do they do? Write down your thoughts.

It transpires that Stephen had received inpatient care in a local mental health unit for adolescents. On further enquiry it was established that Stephen had used cannabis from the age of around 12 and had experienced delusions on such use. He says he had been excluded from school for supplying drugs to peers and had been arrested on many occasions in relation to drugs. He had spells of 'living rough' and had been abused by older rough sleepers.

ACTIVITY 9.9

What are delusions and how may they cause risks? Write down your thoughts.

Talking more about his chest pain, Stephen says that is being caused by not using cannabis (something he stopped about three weeks ago, after being thrown out of the family home for problems associated with it by his parents). Stephen admits that he is 'sofa surfing' (which he has done before when asked to leave places) and that he is feeling quite tense. This tension is often expressed in losing his temper. Stephen admits to having hit his mother when delusional and after this incident he felt so bad that he took an overdose of paracetamol. The event made him think about his brother's death and he wondered whether he had had any influence on this. He says he doesn't care what happens to him.

ACTIVITY 9.10

What risks do you think Stephen poses to himself and others? Write down your thoughts and try to evaluate how Stephen judges the level of risk to himself and others.

CHAPTER SUMMARY

Key points to take away from *Chapter 9*:
- ☑ Risk is present in all aspects of our own and other people's lives.
- ☑ The general public is portrayed by the media as being in danger from people with mental ill health, yet reports show that the mentally ill are more at risk from the general public.
- ☑ Many of the ways that risk is conceptualised (to self, to others, neglect and vulnerability) are influenced by awareness of the person's history.
- ☑ Risk is not solely dependent on the person but is also influenced by others in society, including the media.
- ☑ Various guidelines highlight safeguarding needs and approaches, and nurses need to be aware of these in order not to exacerbate the risks already facing a person or introduce new risks.
- ☑ Using risk assessment tools is only part of understanding risk; appreciating the other contributory factors and their importance to a person with mental ill health is also essential in assessing the person.

Questions

Question 9.1	Describe how risk is viewed within health care. (*Learning outcome 9.1*)
Question 9.2	Describe the process and elements of assessing risk. (*Learning outcome 9.2*)
Question 9.3	What are the static and dynamic presentations of risk in patients? (*Learning outcome 9.3*)
Question 9.4	Reflect on and detail the factors that may increase the risk of violence and suicide in people with mental health difficulties. (*Learning objectives 9.4 and 9.5*)

FURTHER READING

Hart, C. (2014) *A Pocket Guide to Risk Assessment and Management in Mental Health*. Routledge.

Fitzgerald, N. and Fitzgerald, R. (2016) *Mental Status Examination: a comprehensive core skills guide for all health professionals*. CreateSpace Independent Publishing Platform.

Social Care Institute for Excellence (2015) *Safeguarding Adults Reviews (SARs) under the Care Act*. Available at: www.scie.org.uk/safeguarding/adults/reviews/care-act (accessed 23 June 2021).

Time to Change: www.time-to-change.org.uk

References

Age UK (2019) *Later Life in the United Kingdom*. Age UK.

Ahmedani, B.K., Peterson, E.L., Hu, Y. *et al.* (2017) Major physical health conditions and risk of suicide. *American Journal of Preventive Medicine*, **53(3)**: 308–15.

Aked, J., Marks, N., Cordon, C. and Thompson, S. (2008) *Five Ways to Wellbeing*. New Economics Foundation.

Ali, M. (2017) *How to Communicate Effectively in Health and Social Care: a practical guide for the caring professions*. Pavilion Publishing and Media.

Almerie, M.Q., Okba Al Marhi, M., Jawoosh, M. *et al.* (2015) Social skills programmes for schizophrenia. *Cochrane Database of Systematic Reviews*, **6**: CD009006.

Alqam, B.M. (2018) The effects of reminiscence therapy on depressive symptoms among elderly: an evidence based review. *Trauma and Acute Care*, **3(1)**: 1–4.

American Psychiatric Association (2013) *Diagnostic and Statistical Manual of Mental Disorders* (DSM-5) (5th edition). APA.

Angold, A. and Costello, E.J. (2001) 'The epidemiology of disorders of conduct: nosological issues and comorbidity'. In Hill, J. and Maugham, B. (eds) *Conduct Disorders in Childhood and Adolescence*. Cambridge University Press.

Appleby, L. and Wessely, S. (1988) Public attitudes to mental illness: the influence of the Hungerford massacre. *Medicine, Science and the Law*, **28(4)**: 291–5.

Ardito, R. and Rabellino, D. (2011) Therapeutic alliance and outcome of psychotherapy: historical excursus, measurements, and prospects for research. *Frontiers in Psychology*, **2**: 270.

Ashton, C.H. (2001) Pharmacology and effects of cannabis: a brief review. *British Journal of Psychiatry*, **178(2)**: 101–6.

Ashworth, A., Schofield, P. and Das-Munshi, J. (2017) Physical health in severe mental illness. *British Journal of General Practice*, **67(663)**: 436–7.

Avenevoli, S., Swendsen, J., He, J.P. *et al.* (2015) Major depression in the national comorbidity survey–adolescent supplement: prevalence, correlates, and treatment. *Journal of the American Academy of Child & Adolescent Psychiatry*, **54(1)**: 37–44.

Barbui, C., Purgato, M., Abdulmalik, J. *et al.* (2020) Efficacy of psychosocial interventions for mental health outcomes in low-income and middle-income countries: an umbrella review. *The Lancet,* **7(2)**: 162–72.

Barnham, P. and Hayward, R. (1991) *From the Mental Patient to the Person.* Routledge.

Bateman, A. and Holmes, J. (2005) *Introduction to Psychoanalysis: Contemporary Theory and Practice.* Routledge.

Beauchamp, T. and Childress, J. (2019) *Principles of Biomedical Ethics,* 8th edition. Oxford University Press.

Beck, A.T. (1967) *Depression: Causes and Treatment.* University of Pennsylvania Press.

Bell, D. (2006) Inpatient psychotherapy: the art of the impossible. *Psychoanalytic Psychotherapy,* **11(1)**: 3–18.

Beyond Blue (2019) *Mental Health Continuum.* Available at: https://beyou.edu.au/resources/mental-health-continuum (accessed 23 June 2021).

Blashfield, R.K. (1984) *The classification of psychopathology: Neo-Kraepelinian and quantitative approaches.* Plenum.

Bollas, C. (2018) *The Freudian Moment.* Routledge.

Bowlby, J. (1988) *A Secure Base: Clinical applications of attachment theory.* Routledge.

Bradley, J. (1998) 'Confrontation, Appeasement or Communication'. In Anderson, R. and Dartington, A. (eds) *Facing It Out: Clinical Perspectives on Adolescent Disturbance.* Karnac.

Bremner, J. (2002) Neuroimaging of childhood trauma. *Seminars In Clinical Neuropsychiatry,* **7(2)**: 104–12.

Brent, D.A., Johnson, B., Bartles, S. *et al.* (1993) Personality disorder, tendency to impulsive violence, and suicidal behavior in adolescents. *Journal of the American Academy of Child and Adolescent Psychiatry,* **32**: 69–75.

Brooker, C. and Waugh, A. (2013) *Foundations of Nursing Practice: fundamentals of holistic care,* 2nd edition. Elsevier.

Brooks, F., Magnusson, J., Klemera, E. *et al.* (2015) *Health Behaviour in School-Aged Children (HBSC): World Health Organization Collaborative Cross National Study (HBSC England National Report).* University of Hertfordshire.

Brown, S., Inskip, H. and Barraclough B. (2000) Causes of the excess mortality of schizophrenia. *British Journal of Psychiatry,* **177**: 212–17.

Brown, S., Kim, M., Mitchell, C. and Inskip, H. (2010) Twenty-five year mortality of community cohort with schizophrenia. *British Journal of Psychiatry,* **196**: 116–21.

Butler, M., Urosevic, S., Desai, P. *et al.* (2018) *Treatment for Bipolar Disorder in Adults: a systematic review* (Comparative Effectiveness Review no. 208). Agency for Healthcare

Research and Quality (US). Available at: www.ncbi.nlm.nih.gov/books/NBK532183 (accessed 23 June 2021).

Cahoon, G. (2012) Depression in older adults: a nurse's guide to recognition and treatment. *American Journal of Nursing*, **112(11)**: 22–30.

Callahan, D. (2003) Principlism and communitarianism. *Journal of Medical Ethics*, **29**: 287–91.

Care Quality Commission (CQC) (2018) *Mental Health Act: approved mental health professional services.* Available at: www.cqc.org.uk/publications/themed-work/briefing-mental-health-act-approved-mental-health-professional-services (accessed 23 June 2021).

Care Quality Commission (CQC) (2020) *Experts by Experience.* Available at: www.cqc.org.uk/about-us/jobs/experts-experience (accessed 23 June 2021).

Cassedy, P. (2014) 'Humanistic theories'. In Stickley, T. and Wright, N. (eds) *Theories for Mental Health Nursing: a guide for practice.* SAGE Publications.

Centre for Mental Health (2017) *The Future of the Mental Health Workforce.* Centre for Mental Health.

Cheeta, S., Halil, A., Kenny, M. *et al.* (2018) Does perception of drug-related harm change with age? A cross-sectional online survey of young and older people. *BMJ Open*, **8(11)**.

Children Act 1989. Available at: www.legislation.gov.uk/ukpga/1989/41 (accessed 23 June 2021).

Children Act 2004. Available at: www.legislation.gov.uk/ukpga/2004/31 (accessed 23 June 2021).

Cloutier, P., Martin, J., Kennedy, A., Nixon, M.K. and Muehlenkamp, J.J. (2010) Characteristics and co-occurrence of adolescent non-suicidal self-injury and suicidal behaviours in pediatric emergency crisis services. *Journal of Youth and Adolescence*, **39(3)**: 259–69.

Cohen, A. and Phelan, M. (2001) The physical health of patients with mental illness: a neglected area. *Mental Health Promotion Update*, **2**: 15–16.

Cole-King, A., Green, G., Gask, L., Hines, K. and Platt, S. (2013) Suicide mitigation: a compassionate approach to suicide prevention. *Advances in Psychiatric Treatment*, **19**: 276–83.

Collishaw, S., Hammerton, G., Mahedy, L. *et al.* (2016) Mental health resilience in the adolescent offspring of parents with depression: a prospective longitudinal study. *The Lancet Psychiatry*, **3(1)**: 49–57.

Copeland, W.E., Wolke, D., Angold, A. and Costello, E.J. (2013) Adult psychiatric outcomes of bullying and being bullied by peers in childhood and adolescence. *JAMA Psychiatry*, **70(4)**: 419–26.

Costello, E.J., Erkanli, A. and Angold, A. (2006) Is there an epidemic of child or adolescent depression? *Journal of Child Psychology and Psychiatry*, **47(12)**: 1263–71.

Coventry, P., Hays, R., Dickens, C. *et al.* (2011) Talking about depression: barriers to managing depression in people with long term conditions in primary care. *BMC Family Practice*, **12(10)**.

Craig, T.K., Garity, P., Power, P. *et al.* (2004) The Lambeth Early Onset (LEO) Team: randomised controlled trial of the effectiveness of specialised care for early psychosis. *BMJ*, **329(7474)**: 1067.

Cutcliffe, J.R., Travale, R. and Green, T. (2018) 'Trauma-informed care: progressive mental health care for the twenty-first century'. In Santos, J. and Cutcliffe, J. (eds) *European Psychiatric/Mental Health Nursing in the 21st Century: a person-centred evidence-based approach*. Springer.

Dautzenberg, G., Lans, L., Meesters, P.D. *et al.* (2016) The care needs of older patients with bipolar disorder. *Aging and Mental Health*, **20(9)**: 899–907.

De Jong, P. and Berg, I.K. (2002) *Interviewing for Solutions*. Brooks/Cole.

Deacon, B.J. (2013) The biomedical model of mental disorder: a critical analysis of its validity, utility, and effects on psychotherapy research. *Clinical Psychology Review*, **33**: 846–61.

Deighton, J., Lereya, S.T., Patalay, P. *et al.* (2018) *Mental Health Problems in Young People, Aged 11 to 14: results from the first HeadStart annual survey of 30,000 children*. CAMHS Press.

Department for Education (2018) *Working Together to Safeguard Children*. Available at: https://assets.publishing.service.gov.uk/government/uploads/system/uploads/attachment_data/file/942454/Working_together_to_safeguard_children_inter_agency_guidance.pdf (accessed 23 June 2021).

Department of Health (2001) *Seeking Consent: working with children*. DoH.

Department of Health (2009) *Best Practice in Managing Risk: principles and evidence for best practice in the assessment and management of risk to self and others in mental health services*. Available at: https://assets.publishing.service.gov.uk/government/uploads/system/uploads/attachment_data/file/478595/best-practice-managing-risk-cover-webtagged.pdf (accessed 23 June 2021).

Department of Health (2011a) *No Health Without Mental Health: a cross-government mental health outcomes strategy for people of all ages*. Available at: https://assets.publishing.service.gov.uk/government/uploads/system/uploads/attachment_data/file/138253/dh_124058.pdf (accessed 23 June 2021).

Department of Health (2011b) *Safeguarding Adults: the role of health service practitioners*. Available at: https://assets.publishing.service.gov.uk/government/uploads/system/uploads/attachment_data/file/215714/dh_125233.pdf (accessed 23 June 2021).

Department of Health (2015) *Mental Health Act 1983: Code of Practice*. The Stationery Office. Available at: https://assets.publishing.service.gov.uk/government/uploads/system/uploads/attachment_data/file/435512/MHA_Code_of_Practice.PDF (accessed 23 June 2021).

Department of Health and Department of Education (2017) *Transforming Children and Young People's Mental Health Provision: a green paper*. Available at: https://assets.publishing.service.gov.uk/government/uploads/system/uploads/attachment_data/file/664855/Transforming_children_and_young_people_s_mental_health_provision.pdf (accessed 23 June 2021).

Di Florio, A., Smith, S. and Jones, I. (2013) Postpartum psychosis. *The Obstetrician and Gynaecologist*, **15(3)**: 145–50.

Dorning, H., Davies, A. and Blunt, I. (2015) *Focus on: People with Mental Ill Health and Hospital Use. Exploring disparities in hospital use for physical healthcare*. The Health Foundation and Nuffield Trust.

Double, D.B. (2003) Can a biomedical approach to psychiatric practice be justified? *Journal of Child and Family Studies*, **12(4)**: 379–84.

Douglas, K.S., Hart, S.D., Webster, C.D. and Belfrage, H. (2013) *HCR-20V3: assessing risk of violence – user guide*. Mental Health, Law, and Policy Institute, Simon Fraser University.

Dowlen, R., Keady, J., Milligan, C. *et al*. (2018) The personal benefits of musicking for people living with dementia: a thematic synthesis of the qualitative literature. *Arts & Health*, **10(3)**: 197–212.

Drinkwater, C., Wildman, J. and Moffatt, S. (2019) Social prescribing. *BMJ*, **364**: l1285.

Duffin, C. (2016) Assessing the benefits of social prescribing. *Cancer Nursing Practice*, **15(2)**: 18–20.

Ebbesen, M., Andersen, S. and Pedersen, B. D. (2012) Further development of Beauchamp and Childress' theory based on empirical ethics. *Journal of Clinical Research & Bioethics*, **S6**: e001.

Egan, G. (1975) *The Skilled Helper: a systematic approach to effective helping*. Brooks/Cole.

Egede, L.E. and Ellis, C. (2010) Diabetes and depression: global perspectives. *Diabetes Research and Clinical Practice*, **87(3)**: 302–12.

Elliott, D., Bjelajac, P., Fallot, R., Markoff, L. and Glover Reed, B. (2005) Trauma-informed or trauma-denied: principles and implementation of trauma-informed services for women. *Journal of Community Psychology*, **33(4)**: 461–77.

Elliott, R., Bohart, A.C., Watson, J.C. and Greenberg, L.S. (2011) 'Empathy'. In Norcross, J. (ed) *Psychotherapy Relationships That Work*, 2nd edition. Oxford University Press.

Elsabbagh, M., Divan, G., Koh, Y.J. *et al.* (2012) Global prevalence of autism and other pervasive developmental disorders. *Autism Research*, **5(3)**: 160–79.

Engel, G.L. (1977) The need for a new medical model: a challenge for biomedicine. *Science*, **196(4286)**: 129–36.

Faculty of Public Health and Mental Health Foundation (2016) *Better Mental Health For All: a public health approach to mental health improvement.* Faculty of Public Health and Mental Health Foundation. Available at: www.fph.org.uk/media/1644/better-mental-health-for-all-final-low-res.pdf (accessed 23 June 2021).

Fallon, P. (2019) *Madness: a biography.* Red Globe Press.

Fan, Y., Shi, F., Smith, J. *et al.* (2011) Brain anatomical networks in early human brain development. *NeuroImage*, **54(3)**: 1862–71.

Fleet, J. and Ernst, T. (2011) *The Prevention, Recognition and Management of Delirium in Adult In-Patients.* Guy's and St Thomas' NHS Foundation Trust.

Flynn, D. (1998) Psychoanalytic aspects of inpatient treatment. *Journal of Child Psychotherapy*, **24(2)**: 283–306.

Ford, S. (2014) Stress at work makes nurses ill. *Nursing Times,* **110(50)**: 2–3.

Foresight Mental Capital and Wellbeing Project (2008) *Mental Capital and Wellbeing: making the most of ourselves in the 21st century. Final project report.* The Government Office for Science. Available at: https://assets.publishing.service.gov.uk/government/uploads/system/uploads/attachment_data/file/292450/mental-capital-wellbeing-report.pdf (accessed 23 June 2021).

Fowler, D., Hodgekins, J., Howell, L. *et al.* (2009) Can targeted early intervention improve functional recovery in psychosis? A historical control evaluation of the effectiveness of different models of early intervention service provision in Norfolk 1998–2007. *Early Intervention Psychiatry*, **3**: 282–8.

Franks, R. (2016) *Building a Trauma-Informed System of Care for Children in Connecticut.* Available at: www.governor.ct.gov/malloy/lib/malloy/SHAC_Doc_2013.04.26_Franks_presentation.pdf (accessed 23 June 2021).

Freshwater, D. (2005) *Counselling Skills for Nurses, Midwives and Health Visitors*, 2nd edition. Open University Press.

Fung, Y. and Chan, Z. (2011) A systematic review of suicidal behaviour in old age: a gender perspective. *Journal of Clinical Nursing*, **20(15–16):** 2109–24.

Gillon, R. (2003) Ethics needs principles – four can encompass the rest – and respect for autonomy should be 'first among equals'. *Journal of Medical Ethics*, **29**: 307–12.

Goodwin, N. and Lawton-Smith, S. (2010) Integrating care for people with mental illness: The Care Programme Approach in England and its implications for long-term conditions management. *International Journal of Integrated Care*, **10**: E040.

Gray, R., Hardy, S. and Anderson, K. (2009) Physical health and severe mental illness: if we don't do something about it, who will? *International Journal of Mental Health Nursing*, **18**: 299–300.

Greater Manchester Mental Health NHS Foundation Trust (GMMH) (2018) *Reach Beyond and Open Doors Project*. Available at: www.gmmh.nhs.uk/reach-beyond-and-open-doors-project (accessed 23 June 2021).

Greenberg, N., Brooks, S. and Dunn, R. (2015) Latest developments in post-traumatic stress disorder: diagnosis and treatment: Table 1. *British Medical Bulletin*, **114(1)**: 147–55. doi: 10.1093/bmb/ldv014.

Haddad, P. and Haddad, I. (2015) *Mental Health Stigma*. British Association for Psychopharmacology. Available at: www.bap.org.uk/articles/mental-health-stigma (accessed 23 June 2021).

Hammond, J. and Hammond, D. (2019) 'Multidisciplinary work, multidisciplinary team'. In Barrera, A., Attard, C. and Chaplin, R. (eds) *Oxford Textbook of Inpatient Psychiatry*. Oxford University Press.

Hart, C. (2014) *A Pocket Guide to Risk Assessment and Management in Mental Health*. Routledge.

Health Education England (2016) *Social Prescribing at a Glance: North West England. A scoping report of activity for the North West*. Available at: www.hee.nhs.uk/sites/default/files/documents/Social%20Prescribing%20at%20a%20glance.pdf (accessed 23 June 2021).

Health Education England (2021) *The NHS Constitutional Values Hub*. Available at: www.hee.nhs.uk/about/our-values/nhs-constitutional-values-hub-0 (accessed 23 June 2021).

Hennekens, C., Hennekens, A., Hollar, D. and Casey, D. (2005) Schizophrenia and increased risks of cardiovascular disease. *American Heart Journal*, **150(6)**: 115–21.

Heron, J., McGuiness, M., Robertson Blakemore, E., Craddock, N. and Jones, I. (2008) Early postpartum symptoms in puerperal psychosis. *International Journal of Obstetrics and Gynaecology*, **115(3)**: 348–53.

Hippisley-Cox, J., Vinogradova, Y., Coupland, C. and Parker, C. (2007) Risk of malignancy in patients with schizophrenia or bipolar disorder. *Archives of General Psychiatry*, **64(12)**: 1368–76.

Hogg, S. (2013) *Prevention in Mind: all babies count. Spotlight on perinatal mental health*. NSPCC.

Hojat, M., DeSantis, J. and Gonnella, J.S. (2017) Patient perceptions of clinician's empathy: measurement and psychometrics. *Journal of Patient Experience*, **4(2)**: 78–83.

Hong, P., Ilardi, S. and Lishner, D. (2011) The aftermath of trauma: the impact of perceived and anticipated invalidation of childhood sexual abuse on borderline symptomatology. *Psychological Trauma: Theory, Research, Practice, and Policy*, **3(4)**: 360–8.

Hughes, K., Bellis, M.A., Hardcastle, K.A. *et al.* (2017) The effect of multiple adverse childhood experiences on health: a systematic review and meta-analysis. *The Lancet Public Health*, **2(8)**: e356–66.

Human Rights Act 1998. Available at: www.legislation.gov.uk/ukpga/1998/42 (accessed 23 June 2021).

Husk, K., Elston, J., Gradinger, F., Callaghan, L. and Asthana, S. (2019) Social prescribing: where is the evidence? *British Journal of General Practitioners*, **69**: 6–7.

Information Commissioner's Office (2018) *Guide to the General Data Protection Regulation (GDPR)*. Available at: https://assets.publishing.service.gov.uk/government/uploads/system/uploads/attachment_data/file/711097/guide-to-the-general-data-protection-regulation-gdpr-1-0.pdf (accessed 23 June 2021).

Isaacs, A.N., Sutton, K. and Beauchamp, A. (2020) Recovery oriented services for persons with severe mental illness can focus on meeting needs through care coordination. *Journal of Mental Health Policy and Economics*, **23(2)**: 43–8.

Jones-Berry, S. and Munn, F. (2017) One in ten nurse sick days down to stress or depression. *Nursing Standard*, **32(5)**: 12–15.

Jung, N., Wranke, C., Hamburger, K. and Kanuff, M. (2014) How emotions affect logical reasoning: evidence from experiments with mood-manipulated participants, spider phobics and people with exam anxiety. *Frontiers in Psychology*, **5**: 570.

Kendler, K.S. and Jablensky, A. (2011) Kraepelin's concept of psychiatric illness. *Psychological Medicine*, **41(6)**: 1119–26.

Kessler, R.C., Berglund, P., Demler, O. *et al.* (2005) Lifetime prevalence and age-of-onset distributions of DSM-IV disorders in the National Comorbidity Survey Replication. *Archives of General Psychiatry*, **62(6)**: 593–602.

Kezelman, C. and Stavropoulos, P. (2012) *'The Last Frontier': practice guidelines for treatment of complex trauma and trauma informed care and service delivery*. Blue Knot Foundation (Adults Surviving Child Abuse).

Kiesler, D.J. (2000) *Beyond the Disease Model of Mental Disorders*. Praeger Publishers.

King's Fund (2020) *What is social prescribing?* Available at: www.kingsfund.org.uk/publications/social-prescribing (accessed 23 June 2021).

Kitwood, T. (1997) *Dementia Reconsidered: the person comes first*. Open University Press.

Knaak, S., Mantler, E. and Szeto, A. (2017) Mental illness-related stigma in healthcare: barriers to access and care and evidence-based solutions. *Healthcare Management Forum*, **30(2)**: 111–16.

Knight, M., Bunch, K., Tuffnell, D. *et al.* (eds) on behalf of MBRRACE-UK (2019) *Saving Lives, Improving Mothers' Care: lessons learned to inform maternity care from the UK and*

Ireland Confidential Enquiries into Maternal Deaths and Morbidity 2015–17. National Perinatal Epidemiology Unit, University of Oxford.

Kompus, K., Løberg, E. M., Posserud, M. B. and Lundervold, A. J. (2015) Prevalence of auditory hallucinations in Norwegian adolescents: results from a population-based study. *Scandinavian Journal of Psychology*, **56(4)**: 391–6.

Koychev, I. and Ebmeier, K.P. (2016) Anxiety in older adults often goes undiagnosed. *Practitioner*, **260(1789)**: 17–20.

Krebber, A.M.H., Buffart, L.M., Kleiji, G. *et al.* (2013) Prevalence of depression in cancer patients: a meta-analysis of diagnostic interviews and self-report instruments. *Psycho-Oncology*, **23(2)**: 121–30.

Kubler-Ross, E. and Kessler, D. (2005) *On Grief and Grieving: finding the meaning of grief through the five stages of loss.* Scribner.

Law Commission (2017) *Mental Capacity and Deprivation of Liberty.* Available at: www.lawcom.gov.uk/app/uploads/2017/03/lc372_mental_capacity.pdf (accessed 23 June 2021).

Lemma, A. and Young, L. (2010) 'Working with traumatised adolescents: a framework for intervention'. In Lemma, A. and Patrick, M. (eds) *Off the Couch: contemporary psychoanalytic applications.* Routledge.

Lepping, P., Palmstierna, T. and Raveesh, B.N. (2016) Paternalism v. autonomy – are we barking up the wrong tree? *British Journal of Psychiatry*, **209(2)**: 95–6.

Leucht, S., Cipriani, A., Spineli, L. *et al.* (2013) Comparative efficacy and tolerability of 15 antipsychotic drugs in schizophrenia: a multiple-treatments meta-analysis. *The Lancet*, **382(9896)**: 951–62.

Lingford-Hughes, A.R., Welch, S., Peters, L. and Nutt, D.J. (2012) BAP updated guidelines: evidence-based guidelines for the pharmacological management of substance abuse, harmful use, addiction and comorbidity: Recommendations from BAP. *Journal of Psychopharmacology*, **26(7)**: 899–952.

Local Government Association (2018) *Briefing on Working with Risk for Safeguarding Adults Boards.* Available at: www.local.gov.uk/sites/default/files/documents/25.90%20-%20Briefing%20on%20Working%20with%20Risk%20for%20Safeguarding%20Adults%20Board_03.pdf (accessed 23 June 2021).

Mackley, A. (2019) *Suicide Prevention: policy and strategy (briefing paper number 08221).* House of Commons Library. Available at: https://researchbriefings.parliament.uk/ResearchBriefing/Summary/CBP-8221 (accessed 23 June 2021).

Madge, N., Hewitt, A., Hawton, K. *et al.* (2008) Deliberate self-harm within an international community sample of young people: comparative findings from the Child & Adolescent Self-harm in Europe (CASE) Study. *Journal of Child Psychology and Psychiatry*, **49(6)**: 667–77.

Maisano, M.S., Shonkoff, E.T. and Folta, S.C. (2020) Multiple health behavior change for weight loss: a scoping review. *American Journal of Health Behavior*, **44(5)**: 559–71.

Marmot, M., Allen, J., Boyce, T., Goldblatt, P. and Morrison, J. (2020) *Health Equity in England: the Marmot Review 10 years on*. Institute of Health Equity.

May, R., Cooke, A. and Cotton, A. (2008) 'Psychological approaches to mental health'. In Stickley, T. and Bassett, T. (eds) *Learning about Mental Health Practice*. John Wiley & Sons Ltd.

McDaid, D., Hewlett, E. and Park, A. (2017) *Understanding Effective Approaches to Promoting Mental Health and Preventing Mental Illness*. Organisation for Economic Co-operation and Development (OECD).

McIntyre, R.S., McElroy, S.L., Konarski, J.Z. *et al.* (2007) Substance use disorders and overweight/obesity in bipolar I disorder: preliminary evidence for competing addictions. *Journal of Clinical Psychiatry*, **68**: 1352–7.

McManus, S., Bebbington, P., Jenkins, R. and Brugha, T. (eds) (2016) *Mental Health and Wellbeing in England: adult psychiatric morbidity survey 2014*. NHS Digital.

Mental Capacity Act 2005. Available at: www.legislation.gov.uk/ukpga/2005/9/contents (accessed 23 June 2021).

Mental Health Act 1983. Available at: www.legislation.gov.uk/ukpga/1983/20/contents (accessed 23 June 2021).

Mental Health Foundation (2018) *Depression*. Available at: www.mentalhealth.org.uk/a-to-z/d/depression (accessed 23 June 2021).

Mental Health Foundation (2019) *Mental Health Recovery*. Available at: www.mentalhealth.org.uk/a-to-z/r/recovery (accessed 23 June 2021).

Mental Health Taskforce (2016) *The Five Year Forward View for Mental Health*. NHS England.

Menzies Lyth, I. (1959) 'The functioning of social systems as a defence against anxiety'. In *Containing Anxiety in Institutions. Selected essays (volume 1)*. Free Association Books.

Michie, S., van Stralen, M. and West, R. (2011) The behaviour change wheel: a new method for characterising and designing behaviour change interventions. *Implementation Science*, **6(1)**: 42.

Michie, S., Carey, R.N., Johnston, M. *et al.* (2018) From theory-inspired to theory-based interventions: a protocol for developing and testing a methodology for linking behaviour change techniques to theoretical mechanisms of action. *Annals of Behavioral Medicine*, **52(6)**: 501–12.

Mid Staffordshire NHS Foundation Trust (2013) *Report of the Mid Staffordshire NHS Foundation Trust Public Inquiry: executive summary*. The Stationery Office.

Midgley, N. and Kennedy, E. (2011) Psychodynamic psychotherapy for children and adolescents: a critical review of the evidence base. *Journal of Child Psychotherapy*, **37(3)**: 1–29.

Miller, W.R. and Rollnick, S. (2009) Ten things that motivational interviewing is not. *Behavioural and Cognitive Psychotherapy*, **37(2)**: 129–40.

Miller, W.R. and Rollnick, S. (2012) *Motivational Interviewing: helping people change*, 3rd edition. Guilford Press.

Mind (2013) *Mental health crisis care: physical restraint in crisis*. A report on physical restraint in hospital setting in England. Available at: www.mind.org.uk/media-a/4378/physical_restraint_final_web_version.pdf (accessed 23 June 2021).

Mind (2020) *Antipsychotics (A–Z)*. Available at: www.mind.org.uk/information-support/drugs-and-treatments/antipsychotics-a-z/#.XduwbDP7TIU (accessed 23 June 2021).

Misuse of Drugs Act 1971. Available at: www.legislation.gov.uk/ukpga/1971/38/contents (accessed 23 June 2021).

Mitchell, A.E.P. (2019) Depression and behaviourism: beating the blues with pleasurable activity. *Psychology Review*, **24(3)**: 2–4.

Monahan, J., Steadman, H., Silver, E. *et al.* (2001) *Rethinking Risk Assessment: the MacArthur study of mental disorder and violence*. Oxford University Press.

Moncrieff, J. (2008) *The Myth of the Chemical Cure: a critique of psychiatric drug treatment*. Palgrave Macmillan.

Morgan, A.J., Jorm, A.F. and Mackinnon, A. (2013) Self-help for depression via e-mail: a randomised controlled trial of effects on depression and self-help behaviour. *PLoS ONE*, **8(6)**: E66537.

Morgan, A.J., Reavley, N.J., Ross, A., Too, L.S. and Jorm, A.F. (2018) Interventions to reduce stigma towards people with severe mental illness: systematic review and meta-analysis. *Journal of Psychiatric Research*, **103(2018)**: 120–33.

Morgan, S. (2000) *Clinical Risk Management: a clinical tool and practitioner manual*. The Sainsbury Centre for Mental Health.

Murphy, N., Fatoye, F. and Wibberley, C. (2013) The changing face of newspaper representations of the mentally ill. *Journal of Mental Health*, **22(3)**: 1–12.

Murphy, N. (2015) *The Influence of Media Representations on Mental Health Practitioners*. Available at: https://ethos.bl.uk/OrderDetails.do?uin=uk.bl.ethos.658739 (accessed 23 June 2021).

Murray, L. and Cooper, P.J. (2003) 'The impact of postpartum depression on child development'. In Goodyer, I. (ed.) *Aetiological Mechanisms in Developmental Psychopathology*. Oxford University Press.

Muskett, C. (2014) Trauma-informed care in inpatient mental health settings: a review of the literature. *International Journal of Mental Health Nursing*, **23(1)**: 51–9.

Mutiso, V., Pike, K., Musyimi, C. *et al.* (2019) Feasibility of WHO mhGAP-intervention guide in reducing experienced discrimination in people with mental disorders: a pilot study in a rural Kenyan setting. *Epidemiology and Psychiatric Sciences*, **28(2)**: 156–67.

National Clinical Audit of Anxiety and Depression (2019) *How are Inpatient Mental Health Services for People with Anxiety and Depression Performing? Main findings from the National Clinical Audit of Anxiety and Depression: a report co-produced with service users and carers.* Available at: www.hqip.org.uk/wp-content/uploads/2019/10/NCAAD-Main-Report-2019-10-09.pdf (accessed 23 June 2021).

National Collaborating Centre for Mental Health (NCCMH) (2010) *Depression in Adults with a Chronic Physical Health Problem: Treatment and Management.* British Psychological Society. Available at: https://pubmed.ncbi.nlm.nih.gov/22259826/ (accessed 23 June 2021).

National Collaborating Centre for Mental Health (NCCMH) (2012) *Self-harm: Longer-term management.* British Psychological Society and the Royal College of Psychiatrists. Available at: www.nice.org.uk/guidance/cg133/evidence/full-guideline-184901581 (accessed 23 June 2021).

National Collaborating Centre for Mental Health (NCCMH) (2014) *Psychosis and Schizophrenia in Adults: The NICE Guideline on Treatment and Management.* National Collaborating Centre for Mental Health. Available at: www.nice.org.uk/guidance/cg178/evidence/full-guideline-490503565 (accessed 23 June 2021).

National Collaborating Centre for Mental Health (NCCMH) (2018a) *Attention Deficit Hyperactivity Disorder: guidelines on diagnosis management of ADHD in children, young people and adults.* British Psychological Society and Royal College of Psychiatrists. Available at: www.nice.org.uk/guidance/ng87/evidence/full-guideline-pdf-4783651311 (accessed 23 June 2021).

National Collaborating Centre for Mental Health (NCCMH) (2018b) *The Improving Access to Psychological Therapies (IAPT) Pathway for People with Long-term Physical Health Conditions and Medically Unexplained Symptoms: full implementation guidance.* National Collaborating Centre for Mental Health. Available at: www.rcpsych.ac.uk/docs/default-source/improving-care/nccmh/iapt/nccmh-iapt-ltc-full-implementation-guidance.pdf (accessed 23 June 2021).

National Institute for Health and Care Excellence (NICE) (2005) *Obsessive–compulsive Disorder and Body Dysmorphic Disorder: Treatment (CG31).* Available at: www.nice.org.uk/guidance/cg31 (accessed 23 June 2021).

National Institute for Health and Care Excellence (NICE) (2009) *Depression in Adults: recognition and management (CG90).* Available at: www.nice.org.uk/guidance/CG90 (accessed 23 June 2021).

National Institute for Health and Care Excellence (NICE) (2010) *Alcohol-Use Disorders: prevention (PH24)*. Available at: www.nice.org.uk/guidance/ph24 (accessed 23 June 2021).

National Institute for Health and Care Excellence (NICE) (2011a) Alcohol-use disorders: diagnosis, assessment and management of harmful drinking (high-risk drinking) and alcohol dependence (CG115). Available at: www.nice.org.uk/guidance/cg115 (accessed 23 June 2021).

National Institute for Health and Care Excellence (NICE) (2011b) *Common Mental Health Problems: identification and pathways to care (CG123)*. Available at: www.nice.org.uk/guidance/cg123 (accessed 23 June 2021).

National Institute for Health and Care Excellence (NICE) (2011c) *Self-Harm in Over 8s: longer-term management (CG133)*. Available at: http://guidance.nice.org.uk/CG133 (accessed 23 June 2021).

National Institute for Health and Care Excellence (NICE) (2013a) *Self-Harm (QS34)*. Available at: www.nice.org.uk/guidance/qs34 (accessed 23 June 2021).

National Institute for Health and Care Excellence (NICE) (2013b) *Social Anxiety Disorder: recognition, assessment and treatment (CG159)*. Available at: www.nice.org.uk/guidance/cg159 (accessed 23 June 2021).

National Institute for Health and Care Excellence (NICE) (2014a) *Antenatal and Postnatal Mental Health: clinical management and service guidance (CG192)*. Available at: www.nice.org.uk/guidance/cg192 (accessed 23 June 2021).

National Institute for Health and Care Excellence (NICE) (2014b) *Anxiety Disorders (QS53)*. Available at: www.nice.org.uk/guidance/qs53 (accessed 23 June 2021).

National Institute for Health and Care Excellence (NICE) (2014c) *Psychosis and Schizophrenia in Adults: prevention and management (CG178)*. Available at: www.nice.org.uk/guidance/cg178 (accessed 23 June 2021).

National Institute for Health and Care Excellence (NICE) (2015) *Smoking: reducing and preventing tobacco use (QS82)*. Available at: www.nice.org.uk/guidance/qs82 (accessed 23 June 2021).

National Institute for Health and Care Excellence (NICE) (2017) *Drug Misuse Prevention: targeted interventions (NG64)*. Available at: www.nice.org.uk/guidance/ng64 (accessed 23 June 2021).

National Institute for Health and Care Excellence (2018a) *Obsessive–compulsive disorder*. Available at: https://cks.nice.org.uk/topics/obsessive-compulsive-disorder/ (accessed 23 June 2021).

National Institute for Health and Care Excellence (NICE) (2018b) *Post-traumatic stress disorder (NG116)*. Available at: https://www.nice.org.uk/guidance/ng116 (accessed 23 June 2021).

National Institute for Health and Care Excellence (NICE) (2019a) *Eating disorders*. Available at: https://cks.nice.org.uk/topics/eating-disorders/ (accessed 23 June 2021).

National Institute for Health and Care Excellence (NICE) (2019b) *NICEimpact: mental health*. Available at: www.nice.org.uk/media/default/about/what-we-do/into-practice/measuring-uptake/niceimpact-mental-health.pdf (accessed 23 June 2021).

National Institute for Health and Care Excellence (NICE) (2020a) *Bipolar Disorder: assessment and management (CG185)*. Available at: www.nice.org.uk/guidance/cg185 (accessed 23 June 2021).

National Institute for Health and Care Excellence (NICE) (2020b) *Decision-Making and Mental Capacity Overview*. Available at: https://pathways.nice.org.uk/pathways/decision-making-and-mental-capacity (accessed 23 June 2021).

National Institute for Health and Care Excellence (NICE) (2020c) *Eating Disorders: recognition and treatment (NG69)*. Available at: www.nice.org.uk/guidance/ng69 (accessed 23 June 2021).

National Institute of Mental Health (2020) *Obsessive–Compulsive Disorder: when unwanted thoughts or repetitive behaviors take over*. Available at: www.nimh.nih.gov/health/publications/obsessive-compulsive-disorder-when-unwanted-thoughts-take-over/index.shtml (accessed 23 June 2021).

Naylor, C., Parsonage, M., McDaid, D. *et al.* (2012) *Long-Term Conditions and Mental Health: the cost of co-morbidities*. The King's Fund and Centre for Mental Health. Available at: www.kingsfund.org.uk/publications/long-term-conditions-and-mental-health (accessed 23 June 2021).

NHS (2018) *The Improving Access to Psychological Therapies (IAPT) Pathway for People with Long-Term Physical Health Conditions and Medically Unexplained Symptoms*. Available at: www.england.nhs.uk/wp-content/uploads/2018/03/improving-access-to-psychological-therapies-long-term-conditions-pathway.pdf (accessed 23 June 2021).

NHS (2019) *The NHS Long Term Plan*. Available at: www.longtermplan.nhs.uk/wp-content/uploads/2019/08/nhs-long-term-plan-version-1.2.pdf (accessed 23 June 2021).

NHS (2021) *Mental Capacity Act*. Available at: www.nhs.uk/conditions/social-care-and-support-guide/making-decisions-for-someone-else/mental-capacity-act (accessed 23 June 2021).

NHS Commissioning Board (2012) *Compassion in Practice: nursing, midwifery and care staff. Our vision and strategy*. Available at: www.england.nhs.uk/wp-content/uploads/2012/12/compassion-in-practice.pdf (accessed 23 June 2021).

NHS Confederation (2017) *The Role of the Independent Sector in the NHS: busting the myths*. Available at: www.nhsconfed.org/-/media/Confederation/Files/public-access/Independent-sector_Myth-buster.pdf (accessed 23 June 2021).

NHS Digital (2018) *Mental Health of Children and Young People in England 2017: summary of key findings*. Available at: https://files.digital.nhs.uk/A6/EA7D58/MHCYP%202017%20Summary.pdf (accessed 23 June 2021).

NHS Digital (2019) *Statistics on Drug Misuse, England, 2019*. Available at: https://digital.nhs.uk/data-and-information/publications/statistical/statistics-on-drug-misuse/2019 (accessed 23 June 2021).

NHS Digital (2020) *Statistics on Alcohol, England 2020*. Available at: https://digital.nhs.uk/data-and-information/publications/statistical/statistics-on-alcohol/2020 (accessed 23 June 2021).

NHS Digital (2021) *NHS Workforce Statistics – December 2020 (including selected provisional statistics for January 2021)*. Available at: https://digital.nhs.uk/data-and-information/publications/statistical/nhs-workforce-statistics/december-2020 (accessed 23 June 2021).

NHS England (2014) *The Five Year Forward View*. Available at: www.england.nhs.uk/wp-content/uploads/2014/10/5yfv-web.pdf (accessed 23 June 2021).

NHS England (2017) *Mental Health in Older People: a practice primer*. NHS England. Available at: www.england.nhs.uk/wp-content/uploads/2017/09/practice-primer.pdf (accessed 23 June 2021).

NHS England, National Collaborating Centre for Mental Health and the National Institute for Health and Care Excellence (2016) *Implementing the Early Intervention in Psychosis Access and Waiting Time Standard: Guidance*. Available at: www.nice.org.uk/guidance/cg178/resources/implementing-the-early-intervention-in-psychosis-access-and-waiting-time-standard-guidance-pdf-2487749725 (accessed 23 June 2021).

NHS England and NHS Improvement (2019) *Social prescribing and community-based support: Summary guide*. Available at: www.england.nhs.uk/wp-content/uploads/2020/06/social-prescribing-summary-guide-updated-june-20.pdf (accessed 23 June 2021).

NHS Health Advisory Service (1995) *Together We Stand: the commissioning, role and management of child and adolescent mental health services*. The Stationery Office.

Nuffield Trust (2020) *Hospital admissions as a result of self-harm in children and young people*. Available at: www.nuffieldtrust.org.uk/resource/hospital-admissions-as-a-result-of-self-harm-in-children-and-young-people (accessed 23 June 2021).

Nursing and Midwifery Council (NMC) (2013) *NMC Response to the Francis report: the response of the Nursing and Midwifery Council to the Mid Staffordshire NHS Foundation Trust Public Inquiry report*. NMC.

Nursing and Midwifery Council (NMC) (2018a) *Future Nurse: standards of proficiency for registered nurses*. NMC.

Nursing and Midwifery Council (NMC) (2018b) *The Code: professional standards of practice and behaviour for nurses, midwives and nursing associates.* NMC.

Nutt, D.J., King, L.A. and Phillips, L.D. (2010) Drug harms in the UK: a multicriteria decision analysis. *The Lancet*, **76(9752)**: 1558–65.

Office for National Statistics (ONS) (2019) *Suicides in the UK: 2018 registrations.* Available at: www.ons.gov.uk/peoplepopulationandcommunity/ birthsdeathsandmarriages/deaths/bulletins/suicidesintheunitedkingdom/2018regist rations (accessed 23 June 2021).

Oken, B.S., Chamine, I. and Wakeland, W. (2015) A systems approach to stress, stressors and resilience in humans. *Behavioural Brain Research*, **282**: 144–54.

Oud, M., Mayo-Wilson, E., Braidwood, R. *et al.* (2016) Psychological interventions for adults with bipolar disorder: systematic review and meta-analysis. *British Journal of Psychiatry*, **3**: 213–22.

Patey, A.M., Hurt, C.S., Grimshaw, J.M. and Francis, J.J. (2018) Changing behaviour 'more or less' – do theories of behaviour inform strategies for implementation and de-implementation? A critical interpretive synthesis. *Implementation Science*, **13(1)**: 134.

Patton, G.C., Sawyer, S.M., Santelli, J.S. *et al.* (2016) Our future: a Lancet commission on adolescent health and wellbeing. *The Lancet*, **387(10036)**: 2423–78.

Paulson, J.F. and Bazemore, S.D. (2010) Prenatal and postpartum depression in fathers and its association with maternal depression: a meta-analysis. *Journal of the American Medical Association*, **303(19)**: 1961–9.

Peckham, E., Brabyn, S., Cook, L., Tew, G. and Gilbody, S. (2017) Smoking cessation in severe mental ill health: what works? An updated systematic review and meta-analysis. *BMC Psychiatry*, **17(1)**: 252.

Peplau, H.E. (1952) *Interpersonal Relations in Nursing: a conceptual frame of reference for psychodynamic nursing.* Putnam.

Perkins, A., Ridler, J., Browes, D. *et al.* (2018) Experiencing mental health diagnosis: a systematic review of service user, clinician and carer perspectives across clinical settings. *The Lancet Psychiatry*, **5(9)**: 747–64.

Peterson, C. (2012) 'Psychological approaches to mental illness'. In Scheid, T.L. and Brown, T.N. (eds) *A Handbook for the Study of Mental Health: social contexts, theories and systems*, 2nd edition. Cambridge University Press.

Pilgrim, D. (2019) *Key Concepts in Mental Health,* 5th edition. SAGE Publications.

Pitchforth, J., Fahy, K., Ford, T. *et al.* (2018) Mental health and well-being trends among children and young people in the UK, 1995–2014: analysis of repeated cross-sectional national health surveys. *Psychological Medicine,* **49(8)**: 1275–85.

Porter, R. (1987) *The Social History of Madness.* Weidenfeld & Nicolson.

Prince, M., Knapp, M., Guerchet, M., *et al.* (2014) *Dementia UK: Update*. Available from: www.alzheimers.org.uk/sites/default/files/migrate/downloads/dementia_uk_update.pdf (accessed 23 June 2021).

Prochaska, J.O. and DiClemente, C.C. (1982) Transtheoretical therapy: toward a more integrative model of change. *Psychotherapy: Theory, Research and Practice*, **19**: 276–8.

Public Health England (2015) *A Guide to Community-Centred Approaches for Health and Wellbeing*. PHE.

Public Health England (2017) *Better Care for People with Co-Occurring Mental Health and Alcohol/Drug Use Conditions: a guide for commissioners and service providers*. Available at: https://assets.publishing.service.gov.uk/government/uploads/system/uploads/attachment_data/file/625809/Co-occurring_mental_health_and_alcohol_drug_use_conditions.pdf (accessed 23 June 2021).

Public Health England (2018a) *Making Every Contact Count (MECC): implementation guide to support people and organisations when considering or reviewing MECC activity and to aid implementation*. PHE.

Public Health England (2018b) *Safeguarding and Promoting the Welfare of Children Affected by Parental Alcohol and Drug Use: a guide for local authorities*. PHE.

Public Health England (2019a) *Alcohol: applying All Our Health*. PHE.

Public Health England (2019b) *Dependence and Withdrawal Associated with some Prescribed Medicines: an evidence review*. PHE.

Public Health England (2019c) *Guidance on Wellbeing and Mental Health: applying All Our Health*. PHE.

Public Health England (2020a) *How to Use the ASSIST-Lite Screening Tool to Identify Alcohol and Drug Use and Tobacco Smoking*. PHE.

Public Health England (2020b) *Local Alcohol Profiles for England*. PHE.

Public Health England (2020c) *National Drug Treatment Monitoring System (NDTMS)*. PHE.

Rise, I.V., Haro, J. and Gjervan, B. (2016) Clinical features, comorbidity, and cognitive impairment in elderly bipolar patients. *Neuropsychiatric Disease and Treatment*, **12**: 1203–13.

Robson, D. and Gray, R. (2007) Serious mental illness and physical health problems: a discussion paper. *International Journal of Nursing Studies*, **44(3)**: 457–66.

Rogers, C. R. (1957) The necessary and sufficient conditions of therapeutic personality change. *Journal of Consulting Psychology*, **21**: 95–103.

Rollnick, S., Miller, W., Butler, C. and Aloia, M. (2008) Motivational interviewing in health care: helping patients change behavior. *COPD: Journal of Chronic Obstructive Pulmonary Disease*, **5(3)**: 203.

Ross, L.E. and McLean, L.M. (2006) Anxiety disorders during pregnancy and the postpartum period: a systematic review. *Clinical Psychiatry*, **67(8)**: 1285–98.

Royal College of Nursing (2013) *The Independent Sector: history and role in England*. RCN. Available at: www.rcn.org.uk/about-us/our-influencing-work/policy-briefings/POL-3113 (accessed 23 June 2021).

Royal College of Nursing (2015) *Stress and You: a guide for nursing staff*. RCN. Available at: www.rcn.org.uk/professional-development/publications/pub-004967 (accessed 23 June 2021).

Royal College of Psychiatrists (RCPsych) (2010) *Role of the Consultant Psychiatrist: leadership and excellence in mental health services (occasional paper OP74)*. RCPsych.

Royal College of Psychiatrists (RCPsych) (2015) *Perinatal Mental Health Services: recommendations for the provision of services for childbearing women (College report CR197)*. Available at: www.rcpsych.ac.uk/docs/default-source/improving-care/better-mh-policy/college-reports/college-report-cr197.pdf (accessed 23 June 2021).

Royal College of Psychiatrists (RCPsych) (2016) *Rethinking Risk to Others in Mental Health Services (College report CR201)*. Available at: www.rcpsych.ac.uk/docs/default-source/improving-care/better-mh-policy/college-reports/college-report-cr201.pdf (accessed 23 June 2021).

Royal College of Psychiatrists (RCPsych) (2018) *Suffering in Silence: age inequality in older people's mental health care*. RCPsych.

Royal College of Psychiatrists (RCPsych) (2019) *Caring for the Whole Person. Physical healthcare of older adults with mental illness: Integration of care (College report CR222)*. RCPsych.

Rubinsztein, J.S., Sahakian, B.J. and O'Brien, J.T. (2019) Understanding and managing cognitive impairment in bipolar disorder in older people. *BJPsych Advances*, **25**: 150–6.

Ryan, P. and Coughlan, B.J. (2011) 'Older adults' experience of loss, bereavement and grief'. In Ryan, P., Coughlan, B.J., Shahid, Z. and Aherne, C. (eds) *Ageing and Older Adult Mental Health: issues and implications for practice*. Routledge.

Safewards (2020) *Interventions*. Available at: www.safewards.net/table/english/interventions (accessed 23 June 2021).

Sage, N., Sowden, M., Chorlto, E. and Edeleanu, A. (2008) *CBT for Chronic Illness and Palliative Care: a workbook and toolkit*. John Wiley & Sons.

Saunders, K., Hawon, K., Fortune, S. and Farrell, S. (2012) Attitudes and knowledge of clinical staff regarding people who self-harm: a systematic review. *Journal of Affective Disorders*, **139(3)**: 205–16.

Scott, D., Arney, F. and Vimpani, G. (2010) 'Think child, think family, think community'. In Arney, F. and Scott, D. (eds) *Working with Vulnerable Families*, 2nd edition. Cambridge University Press.

Shedler, J. (2010) The efficacy of psychodynamic psychotherapy. *American Psychologist*, **65(2)**: 98–109.

Siegel, D. (2012) *Pocket Guide to Interpersonal Neurobiology: an integrative handbook of the mind.* W.W. Norton & Company Ltd.

Simpson, A., Miller, C. and Bowers, L. (2003) Case management models and the care programme approach: how to make the CPA effective and credible. *Journal of Psychiatric and Mental Health Nursing,* **10(4)**: 472–83.

Skinner, B.F. (1938) *The Behavior of Organisms: an experimental analysis.* Appleton-Century.

Skinner, B.F. (1985) Cognitive science and behaviourism. *British Journal of Psychology,* **76(3)**: 291–301.

Social Care Institute for Excellence (2009) *At a Glance 9: think child, think parent, think family.* Available at: www.scie.org.uk/publications/ataglance/ataglance09.asp (accessed 23 June 2021).

Stafford, M., Steventon, A., Thorlby, R. *et al.* (2018) *Understanding the health care needs of people with multiple health conditions.* The Health Foundation. Available at: www.health.org.uk/publications/understanding-the-health-care-needs-of-people-with-multiple-health-conditions (accessed 23 June 2021).

Stark, E.A., Parsons, C.E., Van Hartevelt, T.J. *et al.* (2015) Post-traumatic stress influences the brain even in the absence of symptoms: a systematic, quantitative meta-analysis of neuroimaging studies. *Neuroscience & Behavioural Reviews,* **56**: 207–21.

Steinberg, H., Carius, D. and Fontenelle, L.F. (2017) Kraepelin's views on obsessive neurosis: a comparison with DSM-5 criteria for obsessive–compulsive disorder. *Revista Brasileira de Psiquiatria* **39(4)**: 355–64.

Stewart, D.E., Robertson, E., Dennis, C-L., Grace, S.L. and Wallington, T. (2003) *Postpartum Depression: literature review of risk factors and interventions.* Toronto Public Health.

Stickley, T. (2011) From SOLER to SURETY for effective non-verbal communication. *Nurse Education in Practice,* **11(6)**: 395–8.

Stickley, T. and Freshwater, D. (2008) 'Therapeutic relations'. In Stickley, T. and Bassett, T. (eds) *Learning About Mental Health Practice.* John Wiley & Sons Ltd.

Suris, J.C., Michaud, P.A. and Viner, R. (2004) The adolescent with a chronic condition. Part 1: developmental issues. *Archives of Disease in Childhood,* **89(10)**: 938–42.

Sussex Partnership NHS Foundation Trust (2019) *Public Consultation on Mental Health Plans Launched.* Available at: www.sussexpartnership.nhs.uk/whats-new/public-consultation-mental-health-plans-launched (accessed 23 June 2021).

Sweeney, A., Filson, B., Kennedy, A., Collinson, L. and Gillard, S. (2018) A paradigm shift: relationships in trauma-informed mental health services. *BJPsych Advances,* **24(5)**: 319–33.

Szmukler, G. and Rose, N. (2013) Risk assessment in mental health care: values and costs. *Behavioural Sciences & the Law*, **31(1)**: 125–40.

Tebes, J.K., Champine, R.B., Matlin, S.L. and Strambler, M.J. (2019) Population health and trauma-informed practice: implications for programs, systems and policies. *American Journal of Community Psychology*, **64(3–4)**: 494–508.

Tracy, D.K, Wood, D.M. and Baumeister, D. (2017) Novel psychoactive substances: types, mechanisms of action, and effects. *BMJ*, **356**: I6848.

Trebilcock, J. and Weston, S. (2019) *Mental Health and Offending: care, coercion and control*. Routledge.

Turner, D.T., van der Gaag, M., Karyotaki, E. and Cuijpers, P. (2014) Psychological interventions for psychosis: a meta-analysis of comparative outcome studies. *American Journal of Psychiatry*, **171(5)**: 523–38.

Turp, M. (2002) *Hidden Self-Harm: narratives from psychotherapy*. Jessica Kingsley Publishers.

Turton, W. (2015) 'An introduction to psychosocial interventions'. In Walker, S. (ed.). *Psychosocial Interventions in Mental Health Nursing*. SAGE Publications.

United Nations Convention on the Rights of the Child (UNCRC) (1989) Available at: www.unicef.org.uk/what-we-do/un-convention-child-rights (accessed 23 June 2021).

University of Manchester (2018) *The Assessment of Clinical Risk in Mental Health Services: National Confidential Inquiry into Suicide and Safety in Mental Health*. University of Manchester.

Vallersnes, O.M., Dines, A.M., Wood, D.M. *et al.* (2016) Psychosis associated with acute recreational drug toxicity: a European case series. *BMC Psychiatry*, **16**: 293.

VanderKruik, R., Barreix, M., Chou, D. *et al.* (2017) The global prevalence of postpartum psychosis: a systematic review. *BMC Psychiatry*, **17**: 272.

Velten, J., Bieda, A., Scholten, S., Wannemüller, A. and Margraf, J. (2018) Lifestyle choices and mental health: a longitudinal survey with German and Chinese students. *BMC Public Health*, **18(1)**: 632.

Von Korff, M., Katon, W.J., Lin, E.H.B. *et al.* (2011) Functional outcomes of multi-condition collaborative care and successful ageing: results of randomised trial. *BMJ*, **343**: d6612.

Vuilleumier, P. (2005) How brains beware: neural mechanisms of emotional attention. *Trends in Cognitive Sciences*, **9(12)**: 585–94.

Waddell, M. (2018) *On Adolescence: inside stories*. Routledge.

Weiland, O. (2020) Mission impossible: curing my mental illnesses. *Writing Waves*, **2(16)**. Available at: https://digitalcommons.csumb.edu/writingwaves/vol2/iss2/16 (accessed 23 June 2021).

Wenzel, A. and Kleiman, K. (2015) *Cognitive Behavioural Therapy for Perinatal Distress*. Routledge.

West, R. (2005) Time for a change: putting the transtheoretical (stages of change) model to rest. *Addiction*, **100(8)**: 1036–9.

Whooley, M. and Unützer, J. (2010) Interdisciplinary stepped care for depression after acute coronary syndrome. *Archives of Internal Medicine*, **170(7)**: 585–6.

Wolpert, M., Harris, R., Jones, M. *et al.* (2014) *THRIVE: the AFC-Tavistock model for CAMHS*. CAMHS Press.

Woolard, J. (2010) *Psychology For The Classroom: behaviourism*. Routledge.

Working Group for Improving the Physical Health of People with SMI (2016) *Improving the Physical Health of Adults with Severe Mental Illness: essential actions (OP100)*. Royal College of Psychiatrists.

World Health Organization (1994) *Lexicon of Alcohol and Drug Terms*. WHO.

World Health Organization (2018a) *Global Status Report on Alcohol and Health: 2018*. WHO.

World Health Organization (2018b) *Mental Health: strengthening our response*. Available at: www.who.int/news-room/fact-sheets/detail/mental-health-strengthening-our-response (accessed 23 June 2021).

World Health Organization (2019a) *International Statistical Classification of Diseases and Related Health Problems (ICD): (ICD-11) (release version)*. WHO. Available at: www.who.int/standards/classifications/classification-of-diseases (accessed 23 June 2021).

World Health Organization (2019b) *Mental Disorders*. Available at: www.who.int/en/news-room/fact-sheets/detail/mental-disorders (accessed 23 June 2021).

World Health Organization (2020) *Adolescent Mental Health*. WHO. Available at: www.who.int/news-room/fact-sheets/detail/adolescent-mental-health (accessed 23 June 2021).

World Health Organization and United Nations Office on Drugs and Crime (2020) *International Standards for the Treatment of Drug Use Disorders: revised edition incorporating results of field-testing*. WHO.

Worth, P. and Proctor, C.L. (2020) 'Congruence/incongruence (Rogers)'. In Zeigler-Hill, V. and Shackelford, T.K. (eds) *Encyclopedia of Personality and Individual Differences*. Springer.

Wright, K. and McKeown, M. (2018) *Essentials of Mental Health Nursing*. SAGE Publications.

Zubin, J. and Spring, B. (1977) Vulnerability: a new view on schizophrenia. *Journal of Abnormal Psychology*, **86**: 103–26.

Index